ACKNOWLEDGMENTS

We both thank Peter Workman for being our match-maker, and our editor, Ruth Sullivan, for her steadfast faith in the project and her relentless pursuit of clarity and simplicity in the writing and organization of the material.

Larry Katz wishes to thank Doris Iarovici, his spouse, for her critical insights, advice, and editorial assistance, and Bonnie Kissell, for unflagging administrative support of this project.

Manning Rubin thanks Jane Rubin, for bearing the brunt of his burying himself in the research, writing, and rewriting he has been obsessed with for two years, and for her level-headed observations that helped the book. And he thanks Larry for the voluminous work he has produced in keeping this book alive.

KEEP YOUR BRAIN ALIVE

KEEP YOUR BRAIN ALIVE

83 Neurobic Exercises to Help Prevent Memory Loss and Increase Mental Fitness

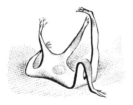

Lawrence C. Katz, Ph.D.
& Manning Rubin

Illustrations by David Suter

Workman Publishing Company, New York

Library of Congress Cataloging-in-Publication Data
Katz, Lawrence C., 1956–
Keep your brain alive: 83 neurobic exercises to help prevent memory loss and increase mental fitness/by Lawrence C. Katz and Manning Rubin.
p. cm.
ISBN-13: 978-0-7611-1052-1; ISBN-10: 0-7611-1052-6
1. Cognition—Age factors. 2. Cognition—Problems, exercises, etc. 3. Memory—Age factors. 4. Cognition—Problems, exercises, etc. 5. Aging—Psychological aspects.
I. Rubin, Manning. II. Title.
BF724.55.C63K38 1999
153—dc21   99-18888
CIP

Workman books are available at special discounts when purchased in bulk for premiums and sales promotions as well as for fund-raising or educational use. Special editions or book excerpts can also be created to specification. For details, contact the Special Sales Director at the address below.

Workman Publishing Company, Inc.
225 Varick Street
New York, NY 10014-4381

Printed in the United States of America

First printing May 1999
20

CONTENTS

PREFACE

As the population of over 76 million Baby Boomers approaches middle age and beyond, the issue of preserving mental powers throughout greatly increased life spans has reached an almost fever pitch. There is a growing interest in—and optimism about—preserving and enhancing the brain's capabilities into senior years. With the help of powerful new tools of molecular biology and brain imaging, neuroscientists around the world have literally been looking into the mind as it thinks. Almost daily, they are discovering that many of the negative myths about the aging brain are, indeed, only myths: "Older and wiser" is not just a hopeful cliché but can be the reality. In much the same way that you can maintain your physical well-being, you can take charge of your mental health and fitness.

Although new and therefore not yet proved by a large body of tests, Neurobics is based on solid scientific ground; it is an exciting synthesis of substantial findings about the brain that provides a concrete strategy for keeping the brain fit and flexible as you grow older.

From Theory to Practice

Jane reached into her pocketbook and fished inside for the keys to her apartment. Usually they were in the out-side flap pocket but not today. "Did I forget them?! No...here they are." She felt their shapes to figure out which one would open the top lock. It took her two tries until she heard the welcome click of the lock opening. Inside the door she reached to the left for the light switch...but why bother? Her husband would do that later. Touching the wall lightly with her fingertips, she moved to the closet on the right, found it, and hung up her coat. She turned slowly and visualized in her mind the location of the table holding her telephone and an-swering machine. Carefully she headed in that direction, guided by the feel of the leather armchair and the scent of a vase of birth-day roses, anxious to avoid the sharp edge of the coffee table and hoping to have some messages from her family waiting.

The table. The answering machine. She reached out and brushed her fingers across what she believed to be the play button. "What if I push the delete button?" she thought, and again checked to make sure she was right. Yesterday it was so easy. She could have done all this simply by looking around. Today was different. She could see nothing.

But Jane had not suddenly gone blind. At age 50, she was introducing a lifestyle strategy called Neurobics into her daily activities. Based on recent discoveries in brain science, Neurobics is a new form of brain exercise designed to help keep the brain agile and healthy. By breaking her usual homecoming routine, Jane had placed her brain's attentional circuits in high gear. With her eyes closed, she had to rely on her senses of touch, smell, hearing, and spatial memory to do something they rarely did—navigate through her apartment. And she was involving her emotional sense by feeling the stresses of not being able to see. All these actions created new and different patterns of neuron activity in her brain—which is how Neurobics works.

This book will explain the principles behind Neurobics and how the exercises enhance the overall health of your brain as you grow older.

NEUROBICS:
The New Science of Brain Exercise

"*What was the name of that actor who was in all the early Woody Allen films? You know…curly brown hair…?*"

The first time you forget the name of a person you should know, a movie title, or an important meeting, you're likely to exclaim—only half-jokingly—"I'm losing it! My brain is turning to Jell-O." Reinforced by messages and images in the mass media, you equate mild forgetfulness with the first stages of accelerating mental decline.

"*…He was just in a Broadway show with, um, what's-her-name. Oh, God, you know who I mean.*"

And maybe they do remember it's Tony Roberts. But if they don't, you become frustrated and preoccupied trying to recall this buried name. Usually beginning in your forties or fifties—sometimes even in your thirties—you start to notice these small lapses: not remembering where you put the car keys or what was on the grocery list you left at home...or being unable to understand the instructions for a new VCR or computer...or forgetting where the car is parked because you left the mall through a different door.

Even though these small lapses don't actually interfere much with daily life, the anxiety they provoke can. You worry that you'll become just like your Aunt Harriet, who can remember details of events from the Depression but not what she did yesterday. Firsthand experiences with people who have difficulty with perception and memory as they age can make you anxious when you suddenly forget something ordinary. No wonder you jump to the conclusion that aging is an inevitable slide into forgetfulness, confusion, or even the first stages of Alzheimer's disease.

The good news, however, is that mild forgetfulness is not a disease like Alzheimer's and action can be taken to combat it. Recent brain research points to new approaches that can be incorporated into everyday activities to develop and maintain brain connections. By adopting these strategies, you may actually enhance your brain's ability to deal with declines in mental agility.

There are numerous myths about the aging brain that neuroscientists are disproving daily. With the help of exciting new technologies, the traditional view of the way the brain ages is being rapidly revised. Evidence clearly shows that the brain doesn't have to go into a steep decline as we get older. In fact, in 1998, a team of American and Swedish scientists demonstrated for the first time that *new brain cells are generated in adult humans.*[1]

Also contrary to popular belief, the mental decline most people experience is not due to the steady death of nerve cells.[2] Instead, it usually results from the thinning out of the number and complexity of *dendrites,* the branches on nerve cells that directly receive and process information from other nerve cells that forms the basis of memory. Dendrites receive information across connections called *synapses.* If connections aren't regularly switched on, the dendrites can atrophy. This reduces the brain's ability to put new information into memory as well as to retrieve old information.

Nerve cells need to keep communicating to stay healthy.

Growing dendrites was long thought to be possible only in the brains of children. But more recent work has shown that *old neurons can grow dendrites to compensate for losses.*[3]

Other experiments show that neural circuits in adult brains have the capacity to undergo dramatic changes—an ability scientists thought was lost after childhood. *The aging brain, however, continues to have a remarkable ability to grow, adapt, and change patterns of connections.*[4]

Discoveries like these are the basis of a new theory of brain exercise. Just as cross training helps you maintain overall physical fitness, Neurobics can help you take charge of your overall mental fitness.

Neurobics aims to help you maintain a continuing level of mental fitness, strength, and flexibility as you age.

The exercise program calls for presenting the brain with nonroutine or unexpected experiences using various combinations of your physical senses—vision, smell, touch, taste, and hearing—as well as your emotional "sense." It stimulates patterns of neural activity that create more connections between different brain areas and causes nerve cells to produce natural brain nutrients, called neurotrophins, that can dramatically increase the size and complexity of nerve cell dendrites.[5] Neurotrophins also make surrounding cells stronger and more resistant to the effects of aging.

Neurobics is very different from other types of brain exercise, which usually involve logic puzzles, memory exercises, and solitary practice sessions that resemble tests. Instead,

Neurobic exercises use the five senses in novel ways to enhance the brain's natural drive to form associations between different types of information. Associations (putting a name together with a face, or a smell with a food, for example) are the building blocks of memory and the basis of how we learn. Deliberately creating new associative patterns is a central part of the Neurobic program.

Putting together the neuroscience findings (pages 6–7) with what scientists already know about our senses led directly to our concept of using the associative power of the five senses to harness the brain's ability to create its own natural nutrients. In short, with Neurobics you can grow your own brain food—without drugs or diet.

The word *Neurobics* is a deliberate allusion to physical exercise. Just as the ideal forms of physical exercise emphasize using many *different muscle groups* to enhance coordination and flexibility, the ideal brain exercises involve activating many *different brain areas* in novel ways to increase the range of mental motion. For example, an exercise like swimming makes the body more fit overall and capable of taking on *any* exercise. Similarly,

THE SCIENTIFIC BASIS FOR NEUROBICS

Neurobics rests on much more than a single breakthrough finding. It is a synthesis of important new information about the organization of the brain, how it acquires and maintains memories, and how certain brain activities produce natural brain nutrients. These findings include:

1. The cerebral cortex, the seat of higher learning in the brain, consists of an unexpectedly large number of different areas, each specialized to receive, interpret, and store information from the senses. What you experience through the senses doesn't all end up in one place in the brain.

2. Connecting the areas of the cerebral cortex are hundreds of different neural pathways, which can store memories in almost limitless combinations. Because the system is so complex and the number of possible combinations of brain pathways so vast, we employ only a small fraction of the possible combinations.

3. The brain is richly endowed with specific molecules—the neurotrophins—which are produced and secreted by nerve cells to act as a kind of brain nutrient that actually promotes the health of these nerve cells as well as the health of their neighbors and the synapses between them.[6]

4. The amount of neurotrophins produced by nerve cells—and how well nerve cells respond to neurotrophins made by other nerve cells—is regulated by how active those nerve cells are. In other words, the more active brain cells are, the more growth-stimulating molecules they produce and the better they respond.[7]

5. Specific kinds of sensory stimulation, especially nonroutine experiences that produce novel activity patterns in nerve cell circuits, can produce greater quantities of these growth-stimulating molecules.[8]

Neurobics makes the brain more agile and flexible overall so it can take on *any* mental challenge, whether it be memory, task performance, or creativity. That's because Neurobics uses an approach based on how the brain works, not simply on how to work the brain.

HOW THE BRAIN WORKS

The brain receives, organizes, and distributes information to guide our actions and also stores important information for future use. The problems we associate with getting older—forgetfulness, not feeling "sharp," or having difficulty learning new things—involve the cerebral cortex and the hippocampus.

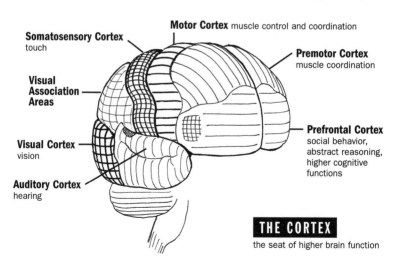

Motor Cortex muscle control and coordination

Somatosensory Cortex
touch

Premotor Cortex
muscle coordination

Visual Association Areas

Prefrontal Cortex
social behavior, abstract reasoning, higher cognitive functions

Visual Cortex
vision

Auditory Cortex
hearing

THE CORTEX

the seat of higher brain function

THE LIMBIC SYSTEM

brain areas involved in processing emotions

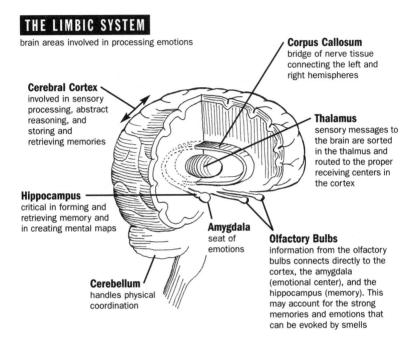

Corpus Callosum
bridge of nerve tissue
connecting the left and
right hemispheres

Cerebral Cortex
involved in sensory
processing, abstract
reasoning, and
storing and
retrieving memories

Thalamus
sensory messages to
the brain are sorted
in the thalmus and
routed to the proper
receiving centers in
the cortex

Hippocampus
critical in forming and
retrieving memory and
in creating mental maps

Amygdala
seat of
emotions

Olfactory Bulbs
information from the olfactory
bulbs connects directly to the
cortex, the amygdala
(emotional center), and the
hippocampus (memory). This
may account for the strong
memories and emotions that
can be evoked by smells

Cerebellum
handles physical
coordination

The cortex is the part of the brain that is responsible for our unique human abilities of memory, language, and abstract thought. The hippocampus coordinates incoming sensory information from the cortex and organizes it into memories. The wiring of the cortex and hippocampus is designed to form links (or associations) between different sensory representations of the same object, event, or behavior.

THE CEREBRAL CORTEX AND HIPPOCAMPUS

Most pictures of the brain usually show the deeply grooved and folded cerebral cortex: a thin sheet of cells (no thicker than twenty pages of this book) wrapped around the other "core" parts of the brain like a rind on a grapefruit. Although thin, the cortex is very large (spread out it would cover the front page of a newspaper) and contains an astounding number of nerve cells—about one hundred million in every square inch. And while the cortex may look like a uniform sheet, it actually consists of dozens, perhaps hundreds, of smaller, specialized regions (some as small as a fingernail, others as large as a credit card). Each of the senses has its own dedicated portions of cortical real estate—for example, there are at least thirty specialized areas just for vision.

Processing information as it comes in from the senses involves a network of many smaller regions. In addition, other regions of the cortex specialize in integrating information from two or more different senses (so, for example, when you hear a sound you know where to look).

These hundreds of regions are linked together by the brain's equivalent of wires: thin threads called axons (each only one hundredth the thickness of a human hair) that extend from nerve cells and conduct electrical impulses from one part of the brain to another. Every cortical region sends and receives millions of impulses via these axons to and from dozens of other cortical regions. The brain contains literally hundreds of miles of such wires. Thus, the cortex resembles an intricate web,

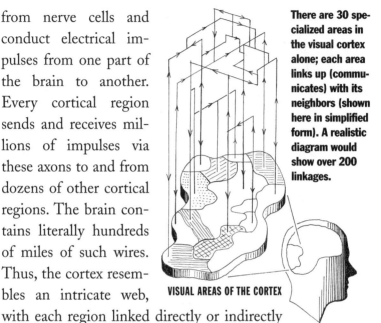

There are 30 specialized areas in the visual cortex alone; each area links up (communicates) with its neighbors (shown here in simplified form). A realistic diagram would show over 200 linkages.

VISUAL AREAS OF THE CORTEX

with each region linked directly or indirectly to many other regions. Some of these connections are between areas that process similar information, such as the thirty involving vision, while other connections are between dissimilar areas, such as touch and smell. The network of pathways between cortical regions that do many different things is what allows the cortex to be so adept at forming associations.

Like the cortex, the hippocampus plays an important role in forming associations. The senses continually flood the brain with information, some of it vital but much of it unimportant. You don't need to remember the face of everyone you pass on the street, but you do want to recognize someone you just met at your boss's party! To prevent the information overload that would accompany having to remember too much, the hippocampus sifts through the barrage of incoming information from the cortex and picks out what to store or discard. In other words, the hippocampus acts like a central clearinghouse, deciding what will be placed into long-term memory, and then, when called upon, retrieving it. The hippocampus's decision to store a memory is believed to hinge on two factors: whether the information has emotional significance, or whether it relates to something we already know.

The hippocampus is also vital for making mental maps, allowing us to remember things like where our car is parked or how to get from home to work. Animals in which the hippocampus has been removed cannot learn or remember simple mazes.

Most problems that cause mental deficiencies involve the cerebral cortex or the hippocampus. So keeping mentally fit really means exercising these parts of our brain so they function at their best. And what they do best is to form associations between different kinds of information they receive.

ASSOCIATIONS: HOW WE LEARN

Associations are representations of events, people, and places that form when the brain decides to link different kinds of information, especially if the link is likely to be useful in the future. The raw material for associations originates primarily from the five senses but also can be emotional or social cues. The brain takes several different things into account in deciding whether to forge these mental connections. For example, if something provides inputs to two or more senses close together in time, like the sight, smell, and taste of a cheeseburger, the brain will almost automatically link the sensations. In essence, this is our basic learning process.

The classic example of associative linking, often taught in introductory psychology courses, is Dr. Ivan Pavlov's experiments with dogs. Dogs normally salivate at the sight of food. Every day when Pavlov fed the dogs, he rang a bell. After a few days, just ringing a bell made the dogs salivate, even if no food was presented.

These dogs made an association—a connection within their brains—that a certain sensory stimulus (the bell) meant food. Consequently, the sound of the bell alone made the brain instruct the salivary glands to get ready for food. Humans and animals can form similar links between almost any kind of sensory inputs.

Obviously, humans are capable of much more sophisticated and abstract learning that isn't as closely tied to external stimuli (like bells) or external rewards (like food). Take learning a language, for example. An infant learns language by associating a particular set of sounds with a certain behavior, person, or object. (An explicit reward may or may not be present.)

Once such associations are formed, they reside in the brain as a long-term memory, which can be accessed just by experiencing the original stimulus. It's rather astounding when you think about it: A certain kind of sensory experience can permanently change the wiring in part of your brain!

Most of what we learn and remember relies on the ability of the brain to form and retrieve associations in much the same way as Pavlov's dogs learned that a bell meant food. For example, you pick up a rose, and its *smell* activates the olfactory (smelling) parts of the cortex, its image activates the *visual* areas, and the soft petals or sharp thorns activate the *feeling* sections. All these different sensations cause nerve cells in very different areas of the cortex to be activated at the same time in a particular pattern, strengthening some of the linkages between these areas.

Once that happens, anything that activates just part of the network will activate all the areas of the brain that have representations of rose events. Someone hands you a rose, and as you hold it, you may remember your first wedding anniversary when you received a dozen roses, which reminds you of your first apartment in that awful building with the broken elevator. Or the smell of roses reminds you of Aunt Harriet's rose garden in late summer where you had picnics with your cousin Arnie who is now living in California and whom you keep meaning to call—all sorts of memories result from a single stimulus.

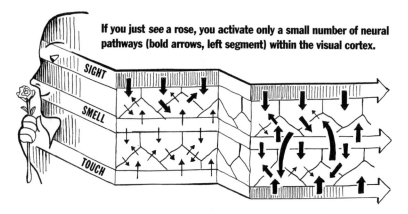

If you just *see* a rose, you activate only a small number of neural pathways (bold arrows, left segment) within the visual cortex.

But if you *smell, touch,* and *see* a rose, a much larger number of direct and indirect pathways *between* the olfactory, visual, and tactile areas are activated (above, right segment). These associative linkages between senses help in memory recall.

MEMORY

Existing programs for brain exercise have ignored this powerful associative route to forming and retrieving memories. Neurobics seeks to access it by providing the cortex with the raw material that will create new and potent associations.

Because each memory is represented in many different cortical areas, the stronger and richer the network of associations or representations you have built into your brain, the more your brain is protected from the loss of any one representation.[1]

Take the common problem of remembering names. When you meet a new person, your brain links a name to a few sensory inputs, such as his appearance (visual). When the brain is younger, these few associations are strong enough so that the next time you see this person, you recall his name. But the more you age, the more people you've met, leaving fewer unique visual characteristics available to represent each new person, so the associative links between visual characteristics and names are more tenuous. Now, imagine closing your eyes in the course of meeting someone. Sensory inputs, other than vision, become much more important as the basis for forming associations necessary for recalling a name: the feel of his hand, his smell, the quality of his voice.

Ordinary First Meeting   **Neurobic First Meeting**

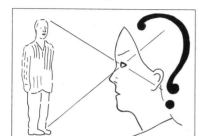 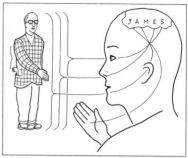

Name Recall: If you use only sight when you meet someone, you're less likely to remember his name. If, on the other hand, you use all your senses, you'll have many more associations—"thinning hair, middle-aged, glasses, hand feels like a damp, limp rag, clothes smell like a smokehouse, voice sounds like a bullfrog"—to recall his name.

You have now tagged someone's name with not just one or two associations, but at least four. If access to one associative pathway is partly blocked ("Gosh, he looks familiar"), you can tap into associations based on other senses and do an end run around the obstruction. Adopting the strategies of forming multisensory associations when the brain is still at or near its peak performance—in the forties and fifties—builds a bulwark against some of the inevitable loss of processing power later in life. If your network of associations is very large, it's like having a very tightly woven net, and the loss of a few threads isn't going to let much fall through.

These multisensory representations for tasks like remembering names were always available to you, but early on, your brain established an effective routine for meeting people that relied primarily on visual cues. An important part of the Neurobic strategy is to help you "see" in other ways—to use other senses to increase the number and range of associations you make. The larger your "safety net," the better your chances of solving a problem or meeting a challenge because you simply have more pathways available to reach a conclusion.

More often than not, adults don't exploit the brain's rich potential for multisensory associations. Think of a baby encountering a rattle. She'll look at it closely, pick it up, and run her fingers around it, shake it, listen to whether it makes a sound, and then most likely stick it in her mouth to taste and feel it with her tongue and lips. The child's rapidly growing brain uses all of her senses to develop the network of associations that will become her memory of a rattle.

Now think of yourself finding a rattle on the floor. Most likely, you'll just look at it and instantly catalog it: "It's a rattle." The point is that a child is constantly tapping into the brain's ability to strengthen and increase connections between its many regions—for smelling, touching, hearing, tasting, and seeing—to produce an ever-growing tapestry of associations…and neural activity.

Adults miss out on this multisensory experience of new associations and sensory involvement because we tend to rely heavily on only one or two senses. As we grow older, we find that life is easier and less stressful when it's predictable. So we tend to avoid new experiences and develop routines around what we already know and feel comfortable with. By doing this, we reduce opportunities for making new

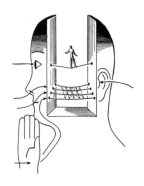

Simultaneous sensory input creates a neural "safety net" that traps information for future access.

associations to a level that is less than ideal for brain fitness.

ROUTINES CAN BE BRAIN-DEADENING

You may be reading this and thinking, "I lead a fairly active life and my brain seems pretty stimulated. Sure, I have my routines, but it's not like I don't see new movies, listen to new songs on the radio, watch TV, or meet new people."

The truth, however, is that most of us go through our adult lives engaged in a series of remarkably fixed routines. Think about your average week…or day-to-day life. Really, how dif-

ferent are your commutes, your breakfasts, lunches, and dinners, week in and week out? And what about things like shopping and laundry? It's startling to realize just how predictable
and free from surprises our everyday lives really are and, as a
consequence, how little we tap into our brain's ability to make
new associations.

Now, routines are not necessarily bad. People created routines because until recent times, the world was unpredictable,
and finding food and shelter was filled with risk and
danger. Once reliable sources of food, water, and shelter were
discovered, it made sense to continue in the same patterns
that allowed them to be obtained with a minimum of risk.
Discovering and practicing successful routines in an
unpredictable world ensured survival.

But in our late-twentieth-century, middle-class American
lives, such unpredictability is largely gone. Food is readily
available at the local supermarket; water flows from the tap;
weather-resistant, heated and cooled houses shrug off the cli-
mate. Modern medicines ward off most common diseases.
We even count on the fact that our favorite TV shows air
each week at the same time.[2]

What consequences does this predictability have on the
brain? Because routine behaviors are almost subconscious,

they are carried out using a minimum of brain energy—*and provide little brain exercise.* The power of the cortex to form new associations is vastly underutilized.

If you drive or walk to work via the same route every day, you use the same brain pathways. The neural links between brain areas required to perform that trip become strong. But other links to areas that were initially activated when the route was novel—such as a new smell, sight, or sound when you rounded a certain corner—get weaker as the trip becomes routine. So you become very efficient at getting from point A to point B, but at a cost to the brain. You lose out on opportunities for novelty and the kind of diverse, multisensory associations that give the brain a good workout.

THE BRAIN HUNGERS FOR NOVELTY

The human brain is evolutionarily primed to seek out and respond to what is unexpected or novel—new information coming in from the outside world that is different from what it expects. It's what turns the brain on. In response to novelty, cortical activity is increased in more and varied brain areas.[3] This strengthens synaptic connections, links different areas together in new patterns, and pumps up production of neurotrophins.

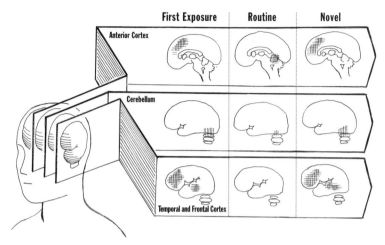

PET scans of three vertical slices of the brain show that significantly more pathways are activated (shown in cross-hatching) when the brain processes a Novel task than when it performs a Routine one. During the routine task (middle column) there is no increased activity in the anterior cortex, cerebellum, or frontal cortex.

But if it is simply *more* activity in the brain that leads to increased neurotrophin production, then listening to more music (even noise), or watching more TV, or getting a massage—all of which stimulate the sense organs—would lead to better brain health. Such passive stimulation of the senses, however, doesn't work as a brain exercise and neither does repeatedly doing the same routine activities. Neurobics is neither passive nor routine. It uses the senses in novel ways to break out of everyday routines.

OUR UNDERUSED SENSES

Our five senses are the portals, or gateways, through which the brain gets its entire contact with the outside world. We rely primarily on our senses of vision and hearing because they quickly tell us a lot about our environment. Our other senses—smell, taste, and touch—are less frequently and obviously called upon. To understand this better, close your eyes and try walking through a room. Instantly, the world around you changes radically. Sounds, smells, and spatial memories of your physical surroundings leap into consciousness. With vision gone, your sense of touch suddenly becomes paramount. Navigating even a familiar environment is a real challenge, and your brain goes into high alert.

The brain has a huge network of pathways based on visual information. That's why so many everyday experiences are geared to visual appeal. In magazine, television, and billboard ads, businesses use visual associations to encourage purchasing decisions. In a world increasingly dominated by shrink-wrapped, plastic-packaged, and deodorized items, the efforts demanded of our other senses, such as touch and smell, are diminished—far more than we're consciously aware of.

Information and associations based on smell used to be

far more relevant than they are today. A keen sense of smell was often vital to survival. Native Americans could track animals by their smell; farmers could smell when a change in the weather was about to happen; smell was important in making sure that foods were safe to eat; doctors even used their sense of smell to diagnose illness. Today, unless you have a very special job, such as creating perfumes, aromas usually function as masks (that's why we use deodorants and fragrances).

Despite its diminished role in our daily lives, however, the sense of smell plays an important role in memory. Associations based on odors form rapidly and persist for a very long time,

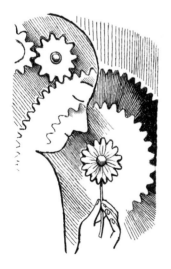

unlike those based on the other senses. The olfactory system is the only sense that has direct connections to the cortex, hippocampus, and other parts of the limbic system involved in processing emotions and storing memories (see illustration, page 10). That's why certain aromas like fresh-baked bread or a particular flower, spice, or perfume can trigger an abundance of emotional responses that

WHAT ABOUT
"SMART DRUGS" AND DIETS?

Progress in neuroscience research has also led to promising drugs for treating serious brain ailments like Alzheimer's and Parkinson's diseases. But an unfortunate by-product of this progress in a society oriented to a "pill for every ill" is a growing demand for medications, pills, or diet supplements that will either magically halt declines in mental abilities or improve performance with a quick fix.

The media perennially tout the promise of new memory-enhancing pills with advertisements for "smart drugs." There are, in fact, drugs that do increase the synaptic transmission in the brain in various ways, and some of these may provide short-term memory enhancements. The problem is that there are always hidden and still unknown risks in using such drugs. (Remember the negative side effects on athletes who took steroids to boost physical performance?) Furthermore, the effects of "smart drugs" are only short term, so they have to be taken continuously.

If, magically, there were a drug to increase mental performance, it would do no good unless you were exercising the brain at the same time. It would be like drinking one of those high-protein boosters and then not doing any physical exercise.

There are also claims that brain performance can be enhanced or preserved by taking large amounts of certain naturally occurring vitamins, minerals, or plant extracts. While there is no question that a well-balanced diet and physical exercise are important for maintaining a healthy brain, there is no clear scientific evidence to support the claimed memory benefits of specific dietary supplements.

We believe a more prudent route to brain health is to harness the brain's ability to manufacture its own natural nutrients. With this approach, neurotrophins and similar molecules will be produced in the right places, and in the right amounts, without side effects.

stimulate the memory of events associated with them. (For example, realtors often advise you to have something delicious baking in the oven when you're showing your house for sale. And if you saw *Scent of a Woman*, you'll remember how Al Pacino's blind character could call up complex associations based on smell alone.)

THE SIXTH SENSE: EMOTION

Researchers are finding that brain circuits for emotions are just as tangible as circuits for the senses, and advanced imaging techniques can now observe this.[4] It is also clear from a number of studies that one's ability to remember something is largely dependent on its emotional context.[5] As we discussed earlier, the hippocampus is more apt to tag information for long-term memory if it has emotional significance. That's why engaging emotions through social interactions is a key strategy of Neurobics.

Interactions with other people are an important trigger of emotional responses. Also, since social situations are generally unpredictable, they are more likely to result in nonroutine activities. Most people have a strong, built-in need for these interactions, and in their absence, mental performance declines.

As we age, our social circles tend to shrink, so an important aspect of Neurobic exercise is to find opportunities to interact with others. Not only does this engage our interest, which directly helps us to remember things, but as the MacArthur Foundation's studies on aging have clearly demonstrated, social interactions themselves have positive effects on overall brain health.[6]

The pace and structure of modern life has reduced the number and intensity of our ordinary, day-to-day social interactions, just as modern conveniences have deprived us of the richness of many sensory stimulations. Remember when buying gas meant talking with an attendant instead of swiping a card at a gas pump? Or getting cash involved dealing with a bank teller instead of pushing buttons on an ATM machine? Or a night out involved going to the movies with a crowd rather than renting a video and sitting alone in front of your VCR? And the computer and the Internet have isolated us even further from any number of personal transactions.

There's ample evidence today that being out in the real world, where you're engaging all the senses, including the important emotional and social "senses," is essential to a healthy brain and an active memory—especially as you age.

■ ■ ■

The aim of Neurobics and the exercises that follow is to provide you with a balanced, comfortable, and enjoyable way to
stimulate your brain.

As we have shown, Neurobics is a scientifically based
program that helps you modify your behavior by introducing
the unexpected to your brain and enlisting the aid of *all* your
senses as you go through your day. An active brain is a
healthy brain, while inaction leads to reduced brain fitness.
Or, in simpler words—"Use it or lose it."

HOW
NEUROBICS
WORKS

There is nothing magic about Neurobics. The magic lies in the brain's remarkable ability to convert certain kinds of mental activity into self-help. Happily for everyone with busy lives, there is no need to find a special time or place to do Neurobic exercises. Everyday life is the Neurobic Brain Gym. Neurobics requires you to do two simple things you may have neglected in your lifestyle: Experience the unexpected and enlist the aid of *all* your senses in the course of the day.

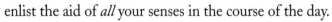

No exercise program is going to help if you aren't motivated and can't find time to do it. That's why Neurobic exercises are designed to fit into what you do on an ordinary day—getting up, commuting, working, shopping, eating, or relaxing. Just as weight-loss experts advise against fad diets in favor of changing your overall eating habits, Neurobics is recommended as a *lifestyle* choice, not a crash course or a quick fix. Simply by making small changes in your daily habits, you can turn everyday routines into "mind-building" exercises. It's like improving your physical state by using the stairs instead of the elevator or walking to the store instead of driving. Neurobics won't give you back the brain of a twenty-year-old, but it can help you to access the vault of memories and experience that a twenty-year-old simply doesn't own. And it can help you keep your brain alive, stronger, and in better shape as you grow older.

Many Neurobic exercises challenge the brain by reducing its reliance on sight and hearing and encouraging the less frequently used senses of smell, touch, and taste to play a more prominent role in everyday activities. By doing so, rarely activated pathways in your brain's associative network are stimulated, increasing your range of mental flexibility.

WHAT MAKES AN EXERCISE NEUROBIC?

Throughout the course of every day, your brain is activated by your senses, and you encounter new stimuli all the time. Why aren't these Neurobic activities? What is it about the specific things we suggest that make them Neurobic?

To begin with, not everything that's novel provides the kind of nerve cell stimulation necessary to activate new brain circuits and enhance neurotrophin production. For example, if you normally write with a pen and one day choose to write everything in pencil, you've broken your routine and are doing something new. But such a small change wouldn't register as an important new sensory association. It would not be enough to engage the circuitry required to really give your brain a workout.

Contrast this with deciding one day to change the hand you normally write with. If you are right-handed, controlling a pen is normally the responsibility of the cortex on the left side of your brain. When you change to writing left-handed, the large network of connections, circuits, and brain areas involved in writing with your left hand, which are normally rarely used, are now activated on the right side of your brain. Suddenly your brain is confronted with a new task that's engaging, challenging, and potentially frustrating.

So, what are the conditions that make an exercise Neurobic? It should do *one or more* of the following:

1. **Involve one or more of your senses in a novel context.**
    By blunting the sense you normally use, force yourself to
    rely on other senses to do an ordinary task. For instance:

    Get dressed for work with your eyes closed.
    Eat a meal with your family in silence.

    Or combine two or more senses in
    unexpected ways:

    Listen to a specific piece of music while
    smelling a particular aroma.

2. **Engage your attention.** To stand out from the back-
    ground of everyday events and make your brain go into
    alert mode, an activity has to be unusual, fun, surprising,
    engage your emotions, or have meaning for you.

    Turn the pictures on your desktop upside down.
    Take your child, spouse, or parent to your office for the day.

3. **Break a routine activity in an unexpected, nontrivial way.**
    (Novelty just for its own sake is not highly Neurobic.)

    Take a completely new route to work.
    Shop at a farmers market instead of a supermarket.

WHAT HAPPENS IN THE BRAIN WITH NEUROBICS

Let's look again at the example on page x of Jane returning home from work and entering her apartment, but now let's consider what is actually happening in her brain that makes these few minutes of her day a Neurobic exercise.

Jane reached into her pocketbook and fished inside for the keys to her apartment. Usually they were in the outside flap but not today. "Did I forget them?! No...here they are." She felt their shapes to figure out which one would open the top lock.

Jane's keys are in the depths of her handbag, which is filled with dozens of different objects—eyeglass case, lipstick, tissues—each with a different texture and shape. Instead of using vision to quickly find the keys, as she might routinely do, she relies now on her sense of *touch*.

Because getting into her apartment is important to her, her brain's attentional and emotional circuits are active as she touches the hard, smooth exterior of her lipstick case, moves past the soft feel of tissues, and eventually identifies the keys. In her brain, long-dormant associations are being reactivated between the areas of her cortex that process touch, areas in the visual part of her cortex that hold the mental "pictures" of objects, and areas of the brain that store the names of objects.

This reactivation causes specific groups of nerve cells to become more active in an unusual pattern for Jane. This in turn can activate the cells' neurotrophin production and strengthen or build another set of connections in her brain's "safety net."

It took her two tries until she heard the welcome click of the lock opening.

Normally, placing a key in a lock uses vision and "motor memory"—an unconscious "map" in the parts of our brain that control movement—which provides an ongoing feedback that allows us to sense where parts of our body are in space. (This is called the proprioceptive sense.) But this time Jane is trying to fit a key into a lock by using the motor map in conjunction with her tactile, not visual, sense. And this nonroutine action is activating and reactivating seldom-used nerve connections between her sense of touch and her proprioceptive sense.

Touching the wall lightly with her fingertips, she moved to the closet on the right, found it, and hung up her coat. She turned slowly and visualized in her mind the location of the table holding her telephone and answering machine

On most days, and in most situations, Jane, like the rest of us, makes her way through the world using sight as a guide. Over time, her visual system has constructed a spatial "map" of her apartment in various parts of the brain. Her other senses of touch and hearing have also been tied into these maps, but these nonvisual connections are rarely called upon. Today, however, Jane is using her sense of touch to trigger a spatial memory of the room in order to navigate through it. The touch pathways that access her spatial maps, usually dormant, are now critically important for accomplishing this simple task and unexpectedly get exercised. And the same holds true for her other senses.

Carefully she headed in that direction, guided by the feel of the leather armchair and the scent of a vase of birthday roses, anxious to avoid the sharp edge of the coffee table and hoping to have some messages from her family waiting.

Here, Jane's olfactory system is kicking into high gear to do something it rarely does—help her smell her way through the world. The olfactory system has a direct line into the hippocampus, the area of the brain that constructs spatial maps of the world. The odor of the roses is working at several brain levels. The emotional association of roses with her birthday, combined with an important emotional goal of getting to her answering machine and retrieving messages from her family, makes them a strong, meaningful stimulus. In addition, Jane is constructing a powerful new association— not only are flowers something that smell good and make you feel good, but they can show you where you are in part of your world.

Today was different...

Yes, it was. By spending just a few minutes doing all the things she normally would do when coming home in a novel way, Jane had engaged literally dozens of new or rarely used brain pathways. Synapses between nerve cells were strengthened by these unusual and challenging activities. And in response to their enhanced activity, some of Jane's brain cells were beginning to produce more brain growth molecules, such as neurotrophins.

Furthermore, as a result of the exercise, a small but significant change has occurred in Jane's brain. New sensory associations, such as the *feel* of the leather armchair, had become part of her brain's vocabulary when she entered the room the next day.

■ ■ ■

HOW TO USE THIS BOOK

Like the body, the brain needs a balance of activities. Fortunately, the ordinary routines present hundreds of opportunities to activate your senses in extraordinary ways. To demonstrate how to incorporate Neurobics into your life, we've taken some "snapshots" of a variety of daily activities. For most of the exercises that follow, we give an explanation (in italics) of what's going on in your brain that makes the exercise work.

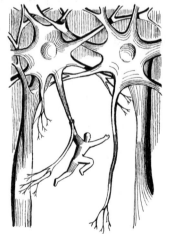

Don't try to use Neurobic exercises for every activity all day long. Instead, pick one or two things from our Neurobic menu: Try "Starting and Ending the Day" today and "Commuting" tomorrow. Mix and match from the various categories so your Neurobic exercises themselves don't become routine. And don't give up those crossword puzzles, reading, learning a new language, travel, engaging with stimulating people, and other kinds of challenging activities that exercise brain circuits in different ways. Once you get the hang of it, we hope you'll begin inventing your own exercises—which is, in itself, Neurobic.

Of course, as with any exercise program, you should be aware of your own physical limitations. And if you have serious concerns about your mental abilities, you should consult a qualified health care professional.

STARTING AND ENDING THE DAY

A ll of us have our morning rituals to get us quickly and "mindlessly" out the door. These set routines allow the brain to go on automatic pilot and be more efficient. And at bedtime, when we need to wind down from a day of mental and physical exertion, routines are similarly comforting.

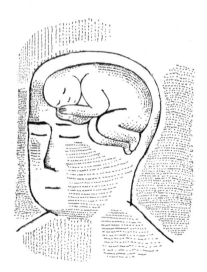

Because routines are so ingrained in our mornings and evenings, they're ideal times to inject a bit of novelty to awaken new brain circuits.

1. WAKE UP AND SMELL THE VANILLA

To change your usual morning olfactory association—waking to the smell of freshly brewed coffee—wake up to something different—vanilla, citrus, peppermint, or rosemary.

Keep an extract of your favorite aroma in an airtight container on your bedside table for a week and release it when you first awaken, and then again as you bathe and dress.

🗩 *Odds are you can't remember specifically when you "learned" to associate the smell of coffee with the start of a day. By consistently linking a new odor with your morning routine, you are activating new neural pathways.*

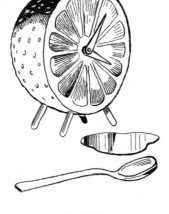

2. SHOWER WITH YOUR EYES CLOSED

Locate the taps and adjust the temperature and flow using just your tactile senses. (Make sure your balance is good before you try this and use common sense to avoid burning or injury.) In the shower locate all necessary props by feel, then wash, shave, and so on, with your eyes shut. Your hands will probably notice varied textures of your own body you aren't aware of when you are "looking."

🗩 *Even though it is probably the least intrusive or time-consuming Neurobic suggestion, this shower exercise will wake up the brain as described in "How Neurobics Works," pages 35–38.*

■ **Variation: Combine Exercises #2 and #4** by laying out your wardrobe the night before (or have someone lay it out for you). Then with your eyes closed, use only tactile associations to distinguish and put on pants, dress, socks, or panty hose, etc.

3. BRUSHING ROULETTE

Brush your teeth with your nondominant hand (including opening the tube and applying toothpaste). You can substitute any morning activity—styling your hair, shaving, applying makeup, buttoning clothes, putting in cuff links, eating, or using the TV remote.

💬 *This exercise requires you to use the opposite side of your brain instead of the side you normally use. Consequently, all those circuits, connections, and brain areas involved in using your dominant hand are inactive, while their counterparts on the other side of your brain are suddenly required to direct a set of behaviors in*

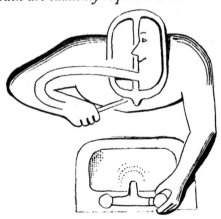

which they usually don't participate. Research has shown that this type of exercise can result in a rapid and substantial expansion of circuits in the parts of the cortex that control and process tactile information from the hand.

Variation: Use only one hand to do tasks like buttoning a shirt, tying a shoe, or getting dressed. For a real workout, try using just your nondominant hand.

Another exercise that associates unusual sensory and motor pathways in your cortex with a routine activity is to use your feet to put your socks and underwear in the laundry basket or pick out your shoes for the day.

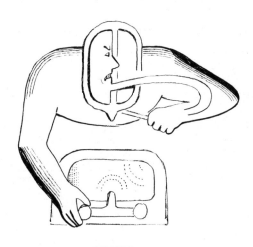

4. A TOUCH OF STYLE

Without looking, choose clothing, shoes, and so on, with matching or contrasting textures. For example, make it a silky, smooth day or a rough, nubby day. Use not only your fingers but also your cheeks, lips, and even your feet—they're all packed with receptors for fine touch.

Extensive practice using the fingers to make fine distinctions between objects or textures causes expansion and rewiring of the brain areas involved in touch. This has been observed in monkeys trained to use their fingers to get food and in brain imaging experiments in blind human Braille readers.

5. SAY WHAT?

Wear earplugs when you join the family for breakfast and experience the world without sound.

💬 *Has your spouse ever complained that you are only "half-listening"? If you're in the middle of a morning routine, it's probably true. By virtue of ingrained routines, your brain has a pretty good idea of what to expect each morning, so only a few words are enough for you to follow a sentence. And, engrossed in a newspaper or listening to the radio, you "tune out" most other sensory inputs. Blocking a major sensory route by wearing earplugs forces you to use other cues to accomplish even simple tasks like knowing when the toast is done or passing the sugar bowl.*

6. Introduce Novelty

We wouldn't recommend trying all these things on the same morning, but do incorporate one or two of the following:

■ Vary the order in which you do your normal routine (e.g., get dressed *after* breakfast).

■ If a bagel and coffee is your daily fare, try something else like hot oatmeal and herbal tea.

■ Change the setting on your radio alarm or tune into a morning TV program you never watch. *Sesame Street,* for example, may arouse the brain to notice how much of what you take for granted is explored in depth by children.

■ Walk the dog on a new route. (Yes, you can teach old dogs new tricks.)

🗩 *Brain imaging studies show that novel tasks activate large areas of the cortex, indicating increased levels of brain activity in several distinct areas. This activity declined when the task had become routine and automatic. Much greater "brain power" is exerted for novel verses automatic (rote) tasks.*

7. CREATE A SENSORY SYMPHONY IN THE BATH

At the end of the day, when you want to wind down, try something relaxing *and* Neurobic, such as a warm bath. Use a variety of sensory stimuli—aromatic bath oils and soaps, sponges, loofah, body scrubs, candlelight, champagne or tea, music, plush towels, and moisturizer. Luxuriate in a cavalcade of scents, textures, and lighting to create linkages between old and new associations.

🗨 *Certain odors evoke distinct moods (alertness, calmness, etc.) in many people. In a Neurobic bath, simply by pairing a specific odor and/or music with an enjoyable, relaxing activity, you form a useful stress-relieving association that can be tapped simply by smelling the aroma or hearing the melody again.*

8. AURAL PLEASURES

Read aloud with your partner. Alternate the roles of reader and listener. It may be a slow way to get through a book, but it's a good way to spend quality time and gives you something to discuss other than your day at work.

● *When we read aloud or listen to someone reading, we use very different brain circuits than when we read silently. One of the earliest demonstrations of brain imaging clearly showed three distinct brain regions lighting up when the same word was read, spoken, or heard. For example, listening to words activated two distinct areas in the left and right hemispheres of the cortex, while speaking words activated the motor cortex on both sides of the brain as well as another part of the brain called the cerebellum. Just looking at words activated only one area of the cortex in the left hemisphere.*

9. SEX: THE ULTIMATE NEUROBIC WORKOUT

Many of the techniques we've suggested in other sections of this book, like shutting one's eyes to heighten sensation in other senses, are an intuitive part of sexual exploration. Novelty—the thrill of the new—plays a central role in sexual arousal. Especially in a long-term marriage, the challenge (and fun) of lovemaking is finding ways to make each time with one's partner a fresh adventure.

Use your imagination and pull out all the sensory stops…wear silk, strew the bed with rose petals, burn lavender incense, have chilled champagne, massage with perfumed oils, put on a romantic CD…and whatever else turns you on.

🗩 *To think that a good sexual encounter also helps keep the brain alive is almost too good to be true. But it is; more than most "routine activities," sex uses every one of our senses and, of course, engages our emotional brain circuits as well.*

COMMUTING

We use mental maps to navigate through our daily lives. By middle age, we've created hundreds of these maps and can readily recall the layout of rooms in houses where we've lived, street grids in towns, interstate highway networks, and the relationships of countries and continents to each other. Because losing one's sense of place is confusing, or even frightening, the brain devotes a lot of processing power to forming and interpreting these mental maps.

Early Polynesian sailors didn't have AAA TripTiks or global positioning systems. They navigated the Pacific by paying attention to multisensory cues—subtle changes in ocean waves, the smell of the sea, the types of seaweed drifting by, and the feel and direction of the wind. In short, these early explorers had available all the ingredients for Neurobic exercise: an important task, the use of all their senses, and novel associations! Today, the opportunities to exercise our brain by exploring uncharted seas are limited. Most days, our visuospatial abilities are called upon to do something much more ordinary—the daily commute.

Unfortunately, the commute is about as far from Neurobic exercise as you can get. It's predictable, routine, and brain-numbing. We've all had the experience of getting to work and having almost no recollection of how we got there. Most of the ride is spent encased in a cocoonlike environment, shielding us from the sights, sounds, and smells of the outside world, and often from other people as well.

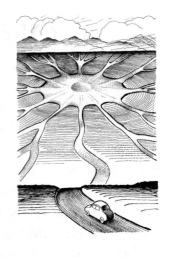

But with a little planning and rethinking, your commuting time can be changed from a passive, mindless activity to one that strengthens the brain. Here are some ideas on how to transform your daily trip into a Neurobic workout.

1. THE SIGHTLESS START

If you drive to work, enter and get ready to start the car with your eyes closed. Using only your sense of touch and spatial memory, find the correct key on your key chain, unlock the car door, slide into the seat, buckle your seatbelt, insert the key into the ignition, and locate familiar controls like the radio and windshield wipers.

🗩 *Just as in the Jane example, on page 35, your tactile sense triggers a spatial memory of where things are via rarely used sets of brain pathways. Closing your eyes also opens up opportunities to form additional associations—like the detailed feel of your keys or the cold steel of the seat-belt buckle—that are suppressed when you rely solely on sight.*

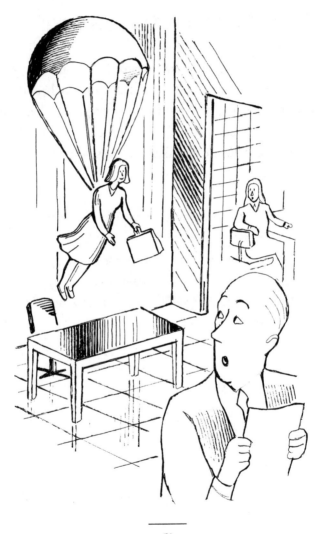

2. BLAZE NEW TRAILS

Take a different route to work. If you're driving, open the windows as in Exercise #4 to help construct a new mental map. If you walk to work, the Neurobic possibilities are even greater.

🗨 *On your routine commute, the brain goes on automatic pilot and gets little stimulation or exercise. An unfamiliar route activates the cortex and hippocampus to integrate the novel sights, smells, and sounds you encounter into a new brain map.*

In one Seinfeld *episode, Kramer is asked how to get to Coney Island from Manhattan. He launches into an elaborate description of subways and buses involving numerous changes scattered throughout the city, various alternatives at each point, and the consequences of each choice. Elaine pipes up and says, "Couldn't you just take the D train straight there?" Well, of course you can. But in this case Kramer was thinking and living "Neurobically," looking for alternative pathways, new possibilities, and engaging his brain's associative powers and navigational abilities to engage in flexible, spatial thinking. Elaine, alas, remains trapped by routine.*

3. FEEL IN CONTROL

Stimulate the tactile pathways involved in the routines of steering, shifting, and signaling by prodding your brain with new materials. (It's important that the new textures be *on* the controls, because that gives the new sensory input importance—you need to drive accurately and skillfully, so you pay attention to anything involved in that process.) Improvise by attaching (with double-stick tape or Velcro) different textures (various grades of sandpaper, for example) to the steering wheel or gear shift. Or buy a few inexpensive steering wheel covers with unusual textures—raised grips, terry cloth, textured vinyl—and use a different one each week.

- Consider swapping cars with a friend who has a very different kind of car (a stick-shift, van, or sport utility vehicle, for example).

- If you're usually the driver, switch and ride in the backseat. Your perspective on the drive will be totally different.

💬 *Different textures produce patterns of activity in the so-matosensory cortex of your brain (that's why you can tell them apart). But after repeated exposure to the same texture, your brain barely pays attention. When you change these textures, driving feels different—and your brain can no longer use familiar assumptions for controlling the car. In addition, using different textures during an activity like driving can activate other association networks in a new context. You might end up describing the morning commute as "rough," not because the traffic was bad, but because that was the tactile stimulus you experienced during the drive.*

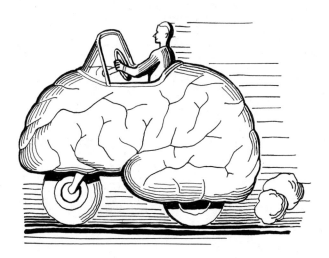

4. WINDOWS OF OPPORTUNITY!

Simply opening the windows as you drive will let in a tapestry of smells—fresh rain on a macadam road, a street vendor's cart, leaves burning in autumn—and sounds—birds singing, kids yelling in a school playground, sirens—that mark your route. Like an ancient navigator, your brain will begin to make and recall associations between the sights, sounds, and odors that you encounter.

Remember that the hippocampus is especially involved in associating odors, sounds, and sights to construct mental maps. Opening the windows provides these circuits with more raw material.

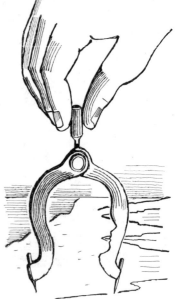

5. TIME TO PUT THE GLOVES ON

Wear work gloves (or heavy mittens) while driving. Blunting your sense of fine touch forces you to rely on other cues to steer the car or change stations on the radio. Caution: Do this only when weather conditions and traffic permit.

🗨 *In addition to fine touch, the skin has receptors for heat, cold, and deep pressure. By blunting fine touch you enhance the role of information coming from pressure receptors and activate different brain pathways involved in driving.*

6. FOLLOW YOUR NOSE

Use odors to form a specific association with a place. Prepare five scent canisters labeled 1 to 5 (see opposite page). At some specific point in your commute—when you pass a certain building, exit, or landmark—open and smell canister #1 for a few seconds to give the place an olfactory "tag." Having created an association between a specific odor and a place, the presence of either the odor or the place will thereafter activate that association. For example, the smell of cloves may call up a mental image or verbal reference of the "big red house" you tagged.

On another day, use another scent canister to "tag" a different place on your route, and so on.

You can do this same exercise while strolling around your neighborhood or walking to work.

🗩 *This exercise creates an olfactory "route map" in your brain, linking the brain areas that help you navigate with the cortical regions that interpret odors. Marrying olfactory associations to places, people, events, or things is also a powerful way to enhance memory.*

MAKING A SCENT CANISTER

Cut an ordinary household sponge into ½-inch cubes. Assemble a variety of different-smelling liquids: for example, vanilla, lemon oil, lavender, cloves, vinegar, or extracts of different flowers or herbs from your own garden or from a health food store. Put a drop or two of liquid on each sponge and place it in a 35 mm film canister. Try to make at least five different canisters.

Leave a canister loosely covered in your car door pocket or cup holder, and open it occasionally for a direct sniff. For a stronger, longer-lasting stimulus, wedge the sponge into the car's air vent. Since some odors linger a long time, be cautious about which ones to use in this way.

7. THE SCENT OF MUSIC

During your drive use aromas to form novel associations between smells and sounds. Instead of using a visual stimulation, this exercise associates auditory stimulation—music—with a specific odor. Start by choosing an odor canister (either deliberately or at random) and a favorite song on a CD or tape. Open the odor canister and take a good sniff every time you listen to that song. Imagine pairing pine odor with a country-western ballad, lavender with the first movement of Beethoven's Sixth Symphony, or cloves with Muddy Waters singing the blues. Be creative with your sound-smell combinations: Try some odd pairings and see what kinds of new associations spring to mind.

🗨 *The goal here is not to remember anything specific, but to provide more raw material to provoke your brain into weaving more associative networks. Both music and smells are powerful stimuli that evoke different emotions. Normally we don't listen to music in the context of odors or vice versa. In this exercise, the repeated pairing of these two stimuli makes your brain create powerful links between the two, increasing the number of pathways available for storing or accessing memories.*

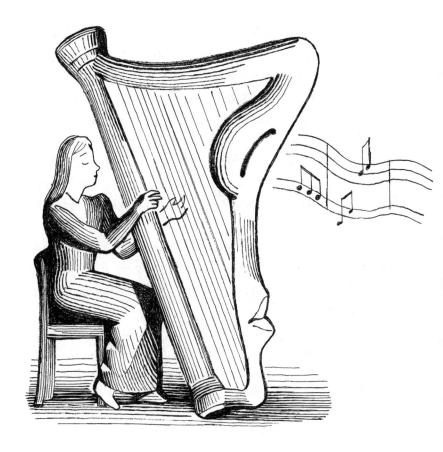

8. THE MIDAS TOUCH

Place a cup filled with different coins in your cup holder. While at a stoplight, try to determine different denominations by feel alone. If your car is equipped with a change holder, place coins into the correct slots, using only your sense of touch.

You can also do this exercise with other small objects of subtly different sizes or textures (various sizes and types of screws, nuts, earrings, or paper clips, 1-inch squares of material such as leather, satin, velour, cotton, or grades of sandpaper). Try to match up a pair of earrings or cuff links, for example.

Because we normally discriminate between objects by looking at them, our tactile discrimination abilities are flabby, like underused muscles. Using touch to distinguish subtly different objects increases activation in cortical areas that process tactile information and leads to stronger synapses. This is the same process that occurs with adults who lose their sight. They learn to distinguish Braille letters because their cortex devotes more pathways to processing fine touch.

9. BE SOCIAL

Don't pass up the many opportunities to enhance the social nature of your commute. Buy the morning or evening paper from a person rather than a vending machine. Need gas? Pay the clerk at the counter rather than just swiping your credit card at the pump.

Wave back and smile or play funny-face games with the kids in the backseat of the car in front of you. Stop at a new place for coffee and a muffin, or a different dry cleaner or flower stand.

💬 *Scientific research has repeatedly proved that social deprivation has severe negative effects on overall cognitive abilities. The ongoing MacArthur Foundation projects validate keeping active socially and mentally as critical factors for mental health.*

10. POOL YOUR THOUGHTS

Along with environmental benefits, car pooling provides opportunities for intimate personal interaction—a form of Neurobic exercise. Four people reading their newspapers in a car pool isn't Neurobic, but using the time to engage with others in lively discussion is. For example, we know of a four-person car pool where each day a different person introduces a subject for discussion—either a controversial topic or provocative story. The rest of the group then reacts.

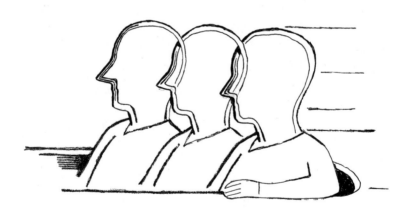

11. LEAVE THE DRIVING TO OTHERS

You can adapt many of the preceding strategies to commuting by bus, train, or even on foot. If you walk to work, take a few different turns. Or get off the bus before or after your usual stop and walk the rest of the way. Take a scent canister and your Walkman and try Exercise #7 on your walk.

On a train or bus, close your eyes and use other cues, such as the speed of the train or bus, or turns in the road, the sound of brakes, or people getting on and off, to visualize where you are and what it looks like outside.

Interact with people around you.

- **Take a still or video camera, or a small sketch pad.** There's a whole world outside the window to record when you're leaving the driving to others.

- **Read something completely different from your normal commuting fare.** Choose a magazine you've never heard of from a newsstand. Read the newspaper classifieds and imagine what you might do with one of the opportunities you see.

AT WORK

Most of us spend about half our waking hours at work. It's also the place where we most fear an obvious loss of cognitive abilities. Our jobs can consume a lot of brain power, but most of that is directed toward specific tasks— generating the next report, fixing a spreadsheet—that don't normally use your brain's associative potential.

While you're busy at work, you don't need logic puzzles or other traditional mental "exercises" to further strain your brain. But you can use Neurobics to give yourself "brain breaks" that stretch and flex your mind throughout the workday.

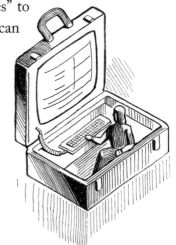

We'll use the example of a desk job and look for the Neurobic opportunities that don't disrupt work efforts or ethics. You may have to tailor these exercises to suit your own work situation.

1. SHAKE THINGS UP A BIT

By using daily exposure and routine, your cortex and hippocampus have constructed a spatial "map" of your desktop so that very little mental effort is required to locate your computer mouse, telephone, stapler, wastebasket, and other office tools. Arbitrarily reposition everything. While you're at it, switch your watch to your other wrist.

🗨 *Scrambling the location of familiar objects you normally reach for without thinking reactivates spatial learning networks and gets your visual and somatosensory brain areas back to work, adjusting your internal maps.*

Moving things around doesn't have to be restricted to your desktop or furniture. If your work schedule is flexible enough, rearrange the order in which you accomplish daily tasks. Do you look at your mail first thing in the morning? Try another time. Can you take your breaks half an hour earlier or later? Or change regularly scheduled meetings from the morning to the afternoon? Within the constraints of your line of work, incorporate a little "disorder."

🗨 *If you want to see the immediate result of rearranging familiar things, simply move your wastebasket from its long-standing position. You'll notice that each time you have something to throw away, you aim at the old spot. The sensory and motor pathways in your brain have been programmed by repeated experience to throw a piece of paper in a certain direction. That moment when you catch yourself and redirect your actions reflects your brain's increased alertness to a novel situation and the beginnings of a new series of instructions being entered into your mental program.*

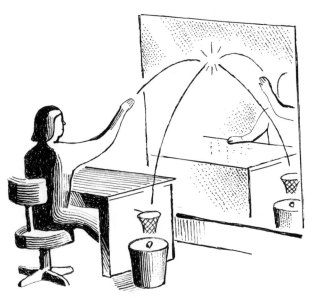

2. SEE THINGS IN A NEW LIGHT

Place different-color gelatin filters (available at art supply or photography stores) over your desk lamp. (Check first for fire hazards).

🗩 *Colors evoke strong emotional associations that can create completely different feelings about ordinary objects and events. In addition, the occasionally odd effects of color (a purple styrofoam coffee cup) jars your brain's expectations and lights up more blips on your attentional "radar screen."*

3. MAKE TASKS ODOROUS

You can activate your memory by pairing an odor and a specific task. For example, to help you remember a certain phone number, use a specific smell every time you dial it. (For this exercise, use the scent canisters described on page 63 or buy a few small herb plants.) Crushing some thyme, mint, or sage provides a strong and effective olfactory cue.

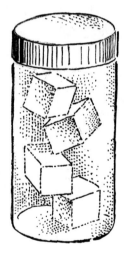

🗩 *Certain odors produce increased alertness and energy. In Japan, nutmeg or cinnamon odors are added to air-conditioning systems of office buildings to enhance productivity. This exercise takes the use of odors one step further: Rather than providing odor stimulation as a passive background to everything you do, odors can be used to highlight specific aspects of your workday, which provides a tag for longer-lasting memory.*

4. LEARN BRAILLE

Most public elevators and ATMs have Braille instructions for blind or visually impaired individuals. In today's world, it's sighted people who suffer "tactile deprivation." Use your fingers to learn the Braille numbers for different floors of your office building or for controlling the elevator doors.

🗨 *When you learned to read, you learned to associate a very specific visual stimulus—a letter or number—with a sound, then with a word, and eventually with meaning. Learning to make distinctions and associations with your fingers—such as between two dots and three dots—activates a whole new set of pathways linking the cognitive regions of your cortex (those parts that know what a letter or number stands for) to the sensory regions. By the time you're able to "read" the button for your floor, using just your fingertips, you'll have built quite a bit of new circuitry in your cortex.*

5. TAKE-SOMEONE-TO-WORK DAY

Bring a friend, child, spouse, or parent to your workplace. Everything you take for granted—the pictures in the halls, the machines you use, your familiar coworkers—are seen anew through another person.

The national Take Our Daughters to Work Day is an excellent example of a novel experience that does wonders not only for your daughter but for your own neural networks.

🗨 *The simple act of making introductions fosters the all-important social interactions that we know are crucial for a healthy brain. Introducing your child (or friend) to coworkers exercises your abilities with names far more effectively than sitting at your desk and trying to memorize them.*

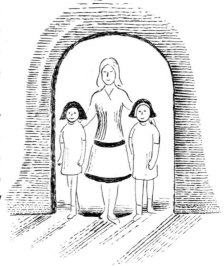

6. THE BRAINSTORM—
AN ASSOCIATION MACHINE

Brainstorming is a very Neurobic activity, because its goal is to encourage individuals to make associations and then to cross-fertilize them with other people's associations.

Arthur B. VanGundy, an expert on brainstorming, suggests having a varied group of four to six people, with one person acting as facilitator and note taker. The facilitator presents the problem or opportunity—whether it's for a new product or service, or resolving a difficult situation. Individuals are encouraged to offer up as many ideas as possible, no matter how unpolished, silly, or "wild." No one may evaluate or judge anything that's brought up, or dominate the session. Instead, participants must free-associate to build or "hitchhike" on each other's suggestions. The facilitator writes the suggestions on a board or sheets of newsprint for all to see and keeps the mood playful and fun. (Afterward, those responsible for the assignment take all the ideas, group them into categories, and select those with the most valuable raw material.)

● *The word* brainstorm *itself conjures up images of flashing lightning bolts. The lightning bolts in the brain are really the electrical flashes crisscrossing between brain areas that only rarely communicate, and the "storm" captures the idea that this exercise provides an environment for increasing the number and intensity of these unusual associations.*

Another effective technique using associations to stimulate creativity is often used by illustrators and art directors. It is based on a technique that originated at the Batelle Institute in Frankfurt, Germany. Write down the assignment or problem, and generate two or more columns of associations that relate to it. Then combine associations from one column with those from the other. If, for example, the task is to illustrate an article about vacations in Alaska, you might list:

Vacations	Alaska
camping	cold
beach	ice
cruise ship	polar bears
camera	eagle
sunglasses	bears
suitcases	salmon
cars, trains, planes	Eskimos
relaxing	oil wells
swimming (pools)	wilderness
eating	snow
sleeping	hunting
reading	fishing
drinks	dog sleds

After much cross-referencing you might decide to illustrate a picture of an Eskimo and a polar bear holding up their salmon to be photographed by a tourist...or a polar bear wearing sunglasses reading in a beach chair and being served drinks.

7. TAKE BRAIN BREAKS

There's more to a coffee break than loading up on caffeine (a short-term brain performance enhancer, actually). Coffee and lunch breaks give you time for mental stretching and social interaction. A brisk fifteen-minute walk outdoors invigorates the body, clears the mind, and opens the door to real-world sensory stimulation. Try fostering nonstressful, mind-expanding interactions during this time. Enlist some coworkers to start a walking, talking, or discussion group during breaks or lunch.

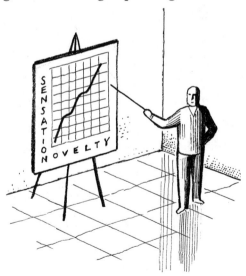

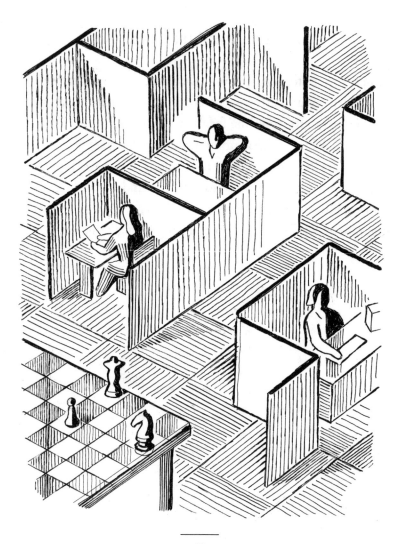

8. ONGOING CHESS GAME

We know of one office where a chessboard was left out near the water cooler. Any employee could come to the board (preferably during a break), assess the situation, and make a move. It was an ongoing game, with no known players, and no winners or losers.

🗩 *Even a novice chess player will weigh dozens of possible moves, attempt to visualize the consequences of each one, then select the move that offers some strategic advantage. This type of "random-player" chess game doesn't allow anyone to develop a long-term strategy. But it does require visual-spatial thinking that is different from what most of us do at work. The brief gear switching provides a break from verbal, left-brain activities and lets the "working brain" take a breather.*

9. TURN YOUR WORLD UPSIDE DOWN

Turn pictures of your family, your desk clock, or an illustrated calendar upside down.

🗨 *Your brain is quite literally of two minds when it comes to processing visual information. The analytical, "verbal" part of your brain (sometimes called the "left brain") tries to label an object after just a brief glance: "table," "chair," "child." The "right brain," in contrast, perceives spatial relationships and uses nonverbal cues. When you look at a familiar picture right side up, your left brain quickly labels it and diverts your attention to other things. When the picture is upside down, the quick labeling strategy doesn't work—and your right-brain networks kick in, trying to interpret the shapes, colors, and relationships of a puzzling picture. The strategy of looking at things upside down is a key component for awakening the latent artist in us, as described by Betty Edwards in* Drawing on the Right Side of the Brain.

10. ADAPT, ADOPT, OR AD LIB

You can adapt many of the exercises from other sections to use in your workplace. For example:

- Get a new cover or cushion for your chair.

- Make a collection of things like small squares of carpet samples, different grades of sandpaper, or different types of paper and tape a few different ones on the underside of your desk or to the side of your computer monitor or phone. Take a few seconds throughout the day to feel each and make fine distinctions between them.

- Collect small objects like paper clips, fasteners, nails, or screws in a cup and during a break or while on the phone, identify them strictly by touch.

- Bring earphones and a portable tape or CD player to use during the workday (or a CD and earphones for your computer). You might experiment with some of the natural environmental tracks available and bring the sea, the surf, the forest, or the jungle into your personal space.

- Try working with the hand you don't normally use for some daily tasks, such as writing, stapling, turning on machines, or dialing the telephone. Or eat your lunch and snacks with the "wrong" hand.

🗨 *As previously discussed, changing which hand you use can unleash a tremendous amount of new brain wiring. You may not think of it as learning, but the nerve cells in your brain do!*

- Change where or with whom you eat lunch. If the weather permits, going outside will almost automatically increase your sensory stimulation compared with staying inside the controlled environment of an office building.

- If you bring your own lunch, you can use many of the ideas from the "At Mealtimes" chapter to make your lunch brain-healthy. One novel example might be to randomly swap brown-bag lunches with a group of coworkers.

AT THE MARKET

For thousands of years getting food was a vigorous, Neurobic workout, involving all the different senses: tracking animals by sight, smell, and sound...deciding when to plant or harvest crops by "reading" the weather...remembering how to locate the best fishing and gathering grounds. Each season presented its own challenges and opportunities for obtaining food, and the fear of going hungry always loomed just over the horizon. Finding food was never routine and it was usually a very social activity. (It is believed that language first originated on the hunt.)

Modern society has effectively eliminated the time, struggle, and unknowns involved in getting food, but we've given up something in exchange for the predictability and convenience of the supermarket. Instead of food being a feast for the senses, supermarket packaging is

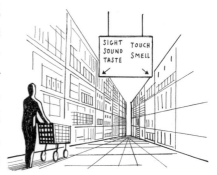

geared to appeal mainly to our visual sense. And in this world of shrink-wrapped, frozen, or canned foods, stimulation based on other senses, such as taste, touch, and smell, are eliminated or relegated to the background. Human exchange has been replaced by automated checkouts, and even the hunting routes (aisles and shelf arrangements) have been preprogrammed for optimum sales, not sensory stimulation.

The exercises in this section attempt to reawaken the hunter-gatherer within, by involving more of your senses and the associations between them, as well as some of the social aspects of the "hunt."

These activities may involve a little extra time (and in some cases, a bit more money), but they have big payoffs in terms of nourishing the brain.

1. Visit a Farmers Market

Since the produce is usually what's available locally and in season, you never know what to expect. Go to the market in an exploratory mode—with no list—and invent a meal from whatever you find that looks, smells, and feels good.

Let's see how a farmers market recruits your senses during apple season. You stop at a farm stand on a fall drive and browse among the varieties of apples available. As you ex-

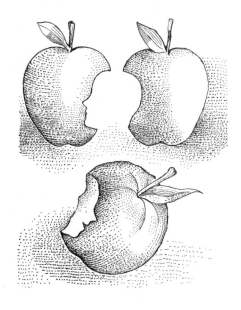

plore the diversity of shapes and colors, pick up an apple of each variety. Feel it for texture and firmness, inhale its aroma. Let the proprietor cut open a Macoun for you to taste, and another apple you've never seen before—an heirloom from his grandfather's orchard that he's been growing for thirty-seven years. You taste the subtle tartness, experience the difference between mealy, juicy, and crisp. Suddenly you are more acutely aware that it's a bright, sunny day, the leaves are changing, there is a smell of fermenting apples in the air, and the sky is a bright blue. Around the one simple act of buying some apples, you have created a rich tapestry of memory.

Chances are the vendors are also the people who grow the apples, and you're sure to encounter some interesting stories and characters. Ask about their farms; this year's crop; and if there's a favorite recipe that uses what you're buying.

🍎 *This exercise ranks high on all the elements of Neurobic requirements: Novelty, multisensory associations between different shapes, colors, smells, and tastes, as well as social interaction.*

2. SHOP AT AN ETHNIC MARKET

An Asian, Hispanic, or Indian market will offer a wide variety of completely novel vegetables, seasonings, and packaged goods depending, of course, on your own ethnic background. Choose a cuisine unfamiliar to you. Ask the storekeepers how to prepare some of the unfamiliar foods on the shelves.

Spend some time in the spices section. Different cultures use radically different seasonings, and you're likely to encounter smells and tastes that you've never experienced.

If you're lucky, the market will have self-serving bins of grains, beans, cereals, and spices. Buy a few small bags of anything that strikes your fancy to use later as tactile, taste, or olfactory stimuli.

The olfactory system can distinguish millions of odors by activating unique combinations of receptors in the nose. (Each receptor is rather like a single note on a piano, while the perception of an odor is like striking a chord.) Encountering new odors adds new chords into the symphony of brain activity. And because the olfactory system is linked directly to the emotional center of the brain, new odors may evoke unexpected feelings and associations, including links to the ethnic group involved.

3. BUTCHER, BAKER, FISHMONGER

You may not have ethnic markets where you live. But most places still have specialty stores staffed by people who know about the products they sell. Ask to see, feel, and smell the merchandise, and about where it came from or how to prepare it. In a fish store, by seeing, feeling, touching, and smelling the catch, you form associative links with the variety of shapes, sizes, and colors.

🗨 *In a bakery, your olfactory sense gets a valuable workout. Certain odors, such as freshly baked bread, trigger emotional responses that stimulate the memory of other events.*

A package of sliced monk-fish looks like a hundred other shrink-wrapped packages, but a whole monkfish—a bizarre, almost grotesque creature—is deeply memorable.

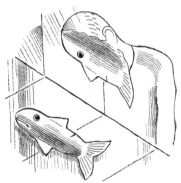

4. PRACTICE NEUROBICS
IN THE SUPERMARKET

- **Use your senses.** Close your eyes and distinguish fruits by their smell or by the feel of their rinds. Use self-serve bins to buy small amounts of grains, cereals, or spices with different tastes, textures, or odors (health food stores are especially good sources).

- **Change your usual route through the aisles.**

- **Ask the people at the meat, fish, or deli counters to help you choose something instead of just picking out prepackaged foods.**

- **Change the way you scan the shelves.** Stores are designed to have the most profitable items at eye level, and in a quick scan you really don't see everything that's there. Instead, stop in any aisle and look at everything displayed on the shelves, from top to bottom. If there's something you've never seen before, pick it up just to read the ingredients and think about it (you don't have to buy it). You've broken your routine and experienced something new.

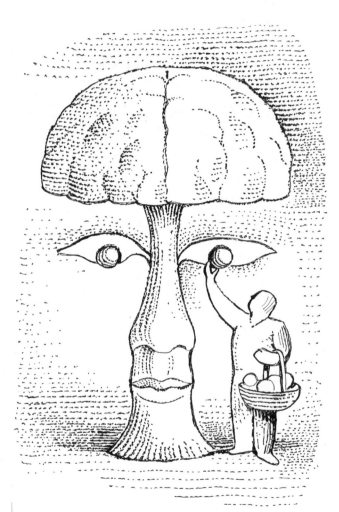

5. REAWAKEN THE HUNTER-GATHERER WITHIN

Each season, you can gather edible plants, fruits, and nuts in the wild—fiddlehead ferns, dandelions, wild asparagus, and grape leaves, various wild berries, mushrooms (careful!), chestnuts, sea wort, wild peas. (If you don't know what things are okay to eat or how to prepare them, take a field guide to edible plants with you on your foraging trips.)

Visit a pick-your-own orchard or farm to gather strawberries, blueberries, corn, or pumpkins. Make the "harvest" a social event by taking along kids or friends.

Another variation is to shop without a list and plan a meal from what looks good at the market that day.

🐚 *Adult brains tend to use the simplest, fastest route to identify objects, while infants and children more often use several senses. Searching for food in the wild prevents the brain from using the easy way out, and hones its ability to make fine discriminations. Is that round green thing a fiddlehead fern (good) or a skunk cabbage sprout (bad)? Without bins, packages, and labels, your brain is forced to pay attention to every cue available in the natural environment.*

6. TREASURE HUNT

Have your spouse or a friend make a list of foods to buy using only descriptors, not the name of the food. For example: "It's about the size and shape of a soccer ball, tannish, heavily veined, dimpled on one end, should feel slightly soft and have a heavy aroma."

🗩 *If one of you makes the list and the other shops for it, you'll both earn Neurobic benefits by tapping into all the sensory association pathways linked to a particular food.*

7. NO MORE ONE-STOP SHOPPING

An old-fashioned hardware store (as opposed to a super-store) is more apt to have employees who really know tools and can talk about how to use them. Instead of being shrink-wrapped, everything—from screws to nuts—can be touched and held. Try stopping in for a Neurobic approach to home improvement.

Or explore a flea market, which ranks high on novelty and the possibilities for social interaction.

Similarly, shopping occasionally at a small bookstore offers more opportunities for genuine social interactions with "book people." You're more likely to encounter recommendations from the staff related to your interests, opening up a whole new reading adventure: "If you like this author, why not try…"

AT MEALTIMES

I n *A Natural History of the Senses,* author Diane Ackerman points out that taste is tightly linked to social activity—the Power Breakfast, celebratory meals, state dinners, ice cream and cake for birthdays, wine and drink for all types of occasions. And since taste is such a sensitive, intimate sense, it is closely linked to emotional memory— think "comfort" food.

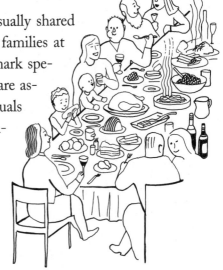

As we grew up, we usually shared the day's events with our families at an evening meal. Foods mark special events in our lives or are associated with religious rituals (the Jewish Seder), or a holiday (Thanksgiving), or a birthday or anniversary.

At meals, our visual, olfactory, tactile, taste, and even our emotional/ pleasure systems are in high gear, feeding associations into our cortex and tapping directly into the most primed memory circuits. Think about it…the sight and feel of silverware, glasses, candlelight…the tastes and textures of bread, finger foods, fried chicken…the tapestry of smells…the sounds of sizzling steaks, clinking glasses, conversation and laughter as well as the emotions that foods evoke…make mealtime potentially a gustatory free-for-all for the senses.

And yet, because it's easier, we tend to make mealtimes predictable and repetitive: We eat the same cereal every morning, the same deli sandwich for lunch, and, if it's Tuesday, meatloaf for dinner. However, mealtimes, more than our other daily activities, offer us the chance to bring all our senses to the table in a pleasurable and brain-healthy way.

Every meal provides an ideal opportunity to engage with spouses, children, friend, or coworkers, and these interactions have demonstrable positive effects on brain health. By changing *how* you eat, without changing *what* you eat, you benefit your brain.

1. MAKE MEALTIMES SOCIAL

Remove the morning paper and other distractions from the breakfast table a few mornings a week and allow your attention to focus on what and with whom you're eating and drinking.

- At dinnertime, turn off the radio or TV and have everyone sit down together. Perhaps start the meal with a prayer or grace that binds people together and links words to food.

🗨 *Remember how teachers used to say, "Let me have your undivided attention"? Neuroscientists studying the brain mechanisms of attention found that it is indeed a limited resource. The more attention you devote to reading a newspaper the less brainpower is available for noticing other things or people in your environment. Of course, keeping up on current events is not bad, but it's worth asking yourself whether you are reading for information or for isolation.*

- At work, organize a brown-bag club where you eat with a group, swap lunches.

- If you live alone, invite a friend for mealtime, even if it's just takeout Chinese. Reinforcing social contacts pays off in brain dividends.

2. SHARE A MEAL IN SILENCE

You'll be surprised at how the foods you taste and the things you hear are greatly enhanced. You'll automatically slow down, savor the food, feel its texture, smell its bouquet, and hear a new ambience that conversation usually smothers.

The absence of verbal communication forces you to use different associative circuits to "speak" and to decipher what's being "said."

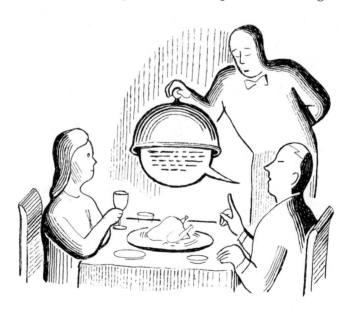

3. MUSICAL CHAIRS

At dinnertime, have everyone switch seats. In most families, everyone has his or her "own" seat, and it's remarkable how permanent these arrangements become. Switching seats changes whose "position" you occupy, who you relate to, your view of the room, and even how you reach for salt and pepper.

🗩 *Like rearranging your desk (page 72), changing your seat at the dinner table provokes "social rearrangements." Each seat has associations attached to it—the kid's seat, the head of the household's seat. Simply by changing places you are challenging and reworking these timeworn associations.*

4. HOLD YOUR NOSE
AS YOU TRY DIFFERENT FOODS

Most of what we call taste actually depends on smell. By closing your nose, you bring basic taste information and tactile cues to the fore and experience the texture and consistency of food using your mouth and tongue.

Taste buds sense sweet, salt, sour or bitter, astringent, and metallic tastes. Your experience of a food based on these qualities, compared to flavor from olfactory stimulation, utilizes different brain pathways.

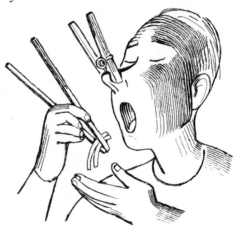

5. PLAN A DEMOCRATIC MEAL

Let each person in the family (even the youngest) decide one item on the menu. Peanut butter and steak may not sound appetizing, but it is not going to hurt you, and it may provide material for some bizarre associations.

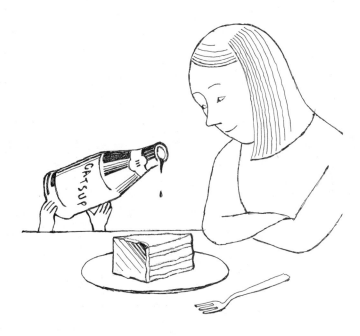

6. A TASTE DOWN MEMORY LANE

Certain foods reactivate and exercise the memory or emotional circuits that were associated with them in the first place. In a memorable passage from *Remembrance of Things Past,* Marcel Proust describes the overwhelming pleasure of childhood memories and associations unleashed by the taste of a madeleine cookie dipped in tea:

At once I had recognized the taste of the crumb of madeleine soaked in her decoction of lime-flowers which my aunt used to give me...immediately the old grey house upon the street, where her room was, rose up like the scenery of a theatre...and with the house the town, from morning to night and in all weathers; the square where I was sent before luncheon, the street along which I used to run errands, the country roads we took when it was fine...so that in that moment all the flowers in our garden and in M. Swann's park, and the water-lilies on the Vivonne and the good folk of the village and their little dwellings and the parish church and the whole of Combray and of its surroundings, taking their proper shapes and growing solid, sprang into being, town and gardens alike, from my cup of tea.

■ Childhood Revisited.

Look for foods that might rekindle childhood memories—a baseball-park hotdog with that neon-yellow mustard, birthday cake and ice cream, Popsicles, s'mores, macaroni and cheese—or any ethnic or regional foods you used to eat as a child and no longer do.

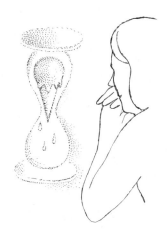

■ The First Bite.

Re-create your first meal with a spouse or lover. Foods you had on a first date or at your wedding can bring back to life long-dormant synapses and provide you with a new route for enhancing past and future memories.

■ Don't Forget the Stuffing.

The foods of Thanksgiving, Passover, Christmas, and the Fourth of July can conjure up all the feelings and memories of holidays past. One taste and, like Proust, you'll be recalling the smell of your grandfather's pipe and your Aunt Rosie telling you not to play under the table. Try creating one of these meals again on a day that's not a holiday.

7. INTRODUCE NOVELTY

- Eat waffles or cereal for dinner. The Norwegians eat their main meal for breakfast. You could try that too.

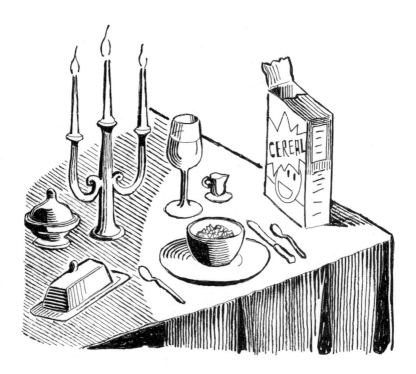

- Change the order in which you eat your food. Try starting with the dessert and ending with the chips. This may seem frivolous but your brain won't think so. It's primed to handle this unexpected strategy.

- Change *where* you eat your meal—a different room, outside, on the porch, on the floor (have an indoor picnic!).

- Puree in a blender one fruit and one vegetable that you have never combined before. Taste it and make up a catchy name for the new concoction. This could be a fun taste game for a group of food lovers.

- Eat your food using your "wrong" hand. A small change like this makes even the most routine acts of eating challenging.

8. SPICE UP YOUR SETTING

Enhance your sensory environment. As we've said, meals are not just about food. Candlelight, visually pleasing china and flowers, beautiful tablecloths, and music provide multisensory stimulation to link with the smells and flavors of food. When you don't have the time or money to indulge, try a new set of place mats or a vase of flowers, or use the good china once in a while—even when you're alone.

🧠 *Enriching the sensory, social, and emotional environment surrounding meals feeds your brain, even though you may not be aware of it at the time. Conversely, when you strip life down to its basics, you deprive your senses. While eating a frozen dinner at a bare table with the TV on satisfies basic caloric needs, it doesn't do much for your olfactory or taste systems, and certainly the emotional impact and novelty factors are low.*

9. FOOD FOR THOUGHT

Mealtimes are also an excellent opportunity to introduce Neurobic stimuli from exotic foods, tastes, and smells:

Once a month try a cuisine that's novel to you. When you eat the same thing at the same time of day, the associative capacity of your smell and taste systems is blunted. So:

- Prepare a breakfast from another country. Here are some typical ones. (The ingredients are generally available at ethnic markets, restaurants, or supermarkets, and finding them can be a Neurobic experience.)

Japan:	seaweed, rice, fish, tea
France:	croissants, cheese, coffee
Mexico:	tortillas and beans
Brazil:	coffee, milk, bread and jam, cheese and ham with papaya
Bulgaria:	Hot platter of eggs or cold platter of eggs, meats, yogurt, honey, bread, and jam

- Try the same thing at dinner. (In cities you can "take out" something.)

  Chinese (and eat with chopsticks!)
  Japanese (chopsticks again)

> Southern fried chicken (eat with your hands)
> Moroccan (eat everything with your fingers)
> Hispanic—Mexican, Brazilian, Spanish (just eat!)

- Accompany the meal with appropriate ethnic music to add an auditory dimension to taste sensations.

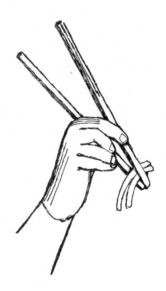

10. CLOSE YOUR EYES AND OPEN WIDE

Identify food on your plate only by smell, taste, and touch. A food's flavor includes its texture, aroma, temperature, spiciness—even sound.

🗩 *Smell and taste, of course, are intimately involved in one's response to foods. But texture plays a role in enjoyment, too, and by isolating your tactile appreciation you create a different neural route. The tongue and lips are among the most sensitive parts of the body (even more sensitive than the fingertips).*

11. HOLD A "BLIND" WINE TASTING

Invite family and/or friends to bring a bottle of a particular kind so that you'll be comparing similar wines. The ritual of a wine tasting involves at least three of your senses. Wine experts judge the color, the aroma, and the taste (sweet, sour, sharp, soft, fruity, heavy, light, complex, oaky, and how it will taste in conjunction with specific foods). Of course, too much tasting can also bring your emotions and sense of balance into play, so be moderate.

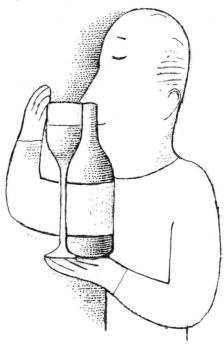

12. NOW YOU'RE COOKIN'

Cook something from scratch. It doesn't have to be a five-course gourmet meal. Making a simple Italian pasta sauce gives all your senses a good workout. As you chop and sauté onions, herbs, and spices, aromas permeate the kitchen and flood you with memories. You're engaging your tactile senses when chopping and peeling, and then in testing the consistency and texture of the sauce as it reduces. A good cook constantly tastes for flavor, adding and adjusting spices a little at a time.

13. HAVE A SEXY MEAL

There was a famous eating scene in the film *Tom Jones,* where the starring couple turn each other on by making each bite highly sensual and suggestive. Stage your own erotic meal with someone you care about and include other sensory enhancements like candles, flowers, music, and incense.

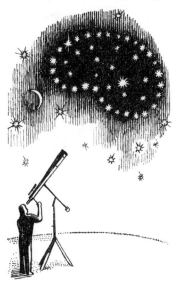

AT LEISURE

Whether it's the end of a long day, a hard week, or a busy month, we all need time to relax and refresh our mind. But not all relaxations are necessarily good for the brain. Watching hours of TV is the most obvious example. Research has shown that watching television literally numbs the mind: The brain is less active during TV-viewing than during sleep! And a constant diet of television is linked to fewer social interactions, which in turn has long-term negative consequences.

In contrast, there are many enjoyable, relaxing activities that incorporate the principles of Neurobics. Some of your existing leisure-time activities are probably more Neurobic and better for your brain than others. So the first step is to take stock of how you spend free time and evaluate whether it includes a good proportion of Neurobics. The key is striking a balance between brain-stimulating Neurobic activity and those times when you simply need to put your mind in idle.

We've grouped exercises into three categories: vacations, leisure time, and hobbies.

1. New Places, New Faces

Throughout this book we've emphasized the importance of breaking routines, and vacation time opens up rich possibilities. Go where you've never been before. Travel broadens, but not if you seek out the McDonald's in Paris or the shopping mall in Santa Fe. Make it a point to explore the visual, auditory, and olfactory differences a new place offers. Sample the local food and entertainment, and shop and travel the way the locals do. Try to avoid traveling in large tour groups, and really get to meet people in different cultures.

🗨 *At every turn, traveling involves something novel for the senses. Spatial maps used for everyday navigation are suddenly unusable and new ones must be constructed. The stress you may feel taking in new sights, sounds, foods, and a foreign language is actually your brain moving into high gear! An afternoon spent talking with the owner of a small shop in a new place may be more memorable (and better for your memory) than going to yet another "must see" sight.*

2. GO CAMP

A camping trip is definitely different from a week by the pool at a resort!

🗩 *There's probably no more di-rect way to experience the unex-pected than camping. Not only are you responsible for constructing your shelter, you have to navigate trails with a compass, make food, and deal firsthand with the chal-lenges of weather and terrain.*

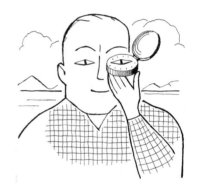

3. A "DO UNTO OTHERS" PROJECT

With your neighbors, get involved in a community project, such as sprucing up a local park. Not only will you interact with kids, neighbors, and the local authorities, but you'll probably use your hands (and brain) in unexpected ways.

4. A DIFFERENT SLANT ON THINGS

If you choose one of these vacations, you'll have contact with people of very different backgrounds and outlooks on the world.

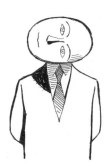

Volunteer as a counselor for a school or scout trip. Volunteer to work for a charity.

Go on an Earthwatch or similar environmental vacation.

If you're a sit-on-the-beach type, consider an active trip—a bicycle tour or a hike on the Appalachian Trail. If you're the hyperactive type, consider a leisurely cruise.

Go to a farm or a dude ranch where vacationers work the farm.

🗩 *The main point is to do something that challenges and engages your mind <u>not because it's difficult</u> but because <u>it's different</u> from what you normally do on vacation.*

5. BE CREATIVE

Take a creative workshop. Lots of places both in the U.S. and abroad offer week- or month-long courses in writing, painting, photography, sculpting, music, acting, archaeology, or whatever you've always wanted to try your hand at.

Try a sports camp. There are "camps" galore, including tennis, golf, scuba diving, riding, baseball, and rock climbing.

Vacation at a cooking school. Your eyes, nose, tongue, sense of touch, and emotions will get an extra workout, and you'll develop mental skills planning, timing, and executing complex tasks.

🗩 *Novelty is the backbone of any good vacation. Increase the Neurobic potential by adding a learning experience to it.*

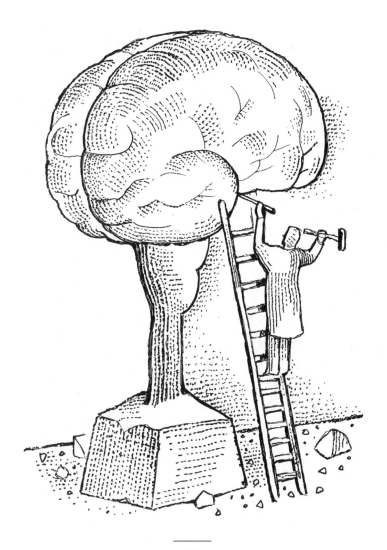

6. THE JOY OF JOY RIDING

Head out without a plan and with family or friends for a "Random Drive." Each passenger gets a turn to suggest where to go or what to do—"Stop here" or "Turn left now" or "Let's wade in that stream!" Or try "Map Toss": Put a map of your region on the floor and have everyone throw a coin on it. Then go to a randomly determined place that strikes your collective fancy. En route, use some of the exercises in the "Commuting" chapter to enhance your social and sensory experiences.

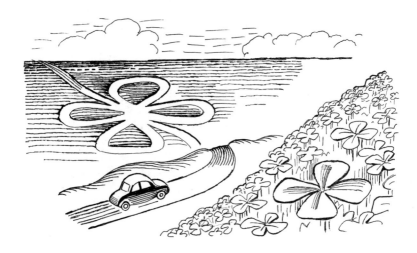

🗨 *Most of the time you're in a car, you have specific destinations in mind (and usually a routine way to get there). Not being sure of what comes next, where you're going to end up, or even how you'll get back turns up your attentional circuits to notice all the new sensory stimuli around you. You (and your passengers) are also exercising spatial navigation skills. And while you can play these games by yourself, by including family and friends you provide opportunities for shared experiences, shared memories, shared meals, and shared associations.*

7. EXPRESS YOURSELF

Do a group art project. Get out drawing paper and crayons or paints and have each person draw something associated with a specific theme (a season, an emotion, or a current event, for example).

Create a mural together on the same paper. For added stimulation, try holding the crayon or paintbrush with your feet instead of your hands.

🗩 *Art is a medium for activating the nonverbal and emotional parts of the cerebral cortex. When you create art, you draw on parts of your brain interested in forms, colors, and textures, as well as thought processes very different from the logical, linear thinking that occupies most of your waking hours.*

8. IMPROV

The visual arts are just one example of using creative expression as a brain exercise.

Dub a segment of a TV show with your own script. Record the show, then play it back without sound. Have each player pick a role and make up dialogue for the part. When everyone is ready, run the tape silently again to your voice-overs. Try the same thing with an animal show like a *National Geographic* special. It's bound to elicit belly laughs.

Play a family video with different kinds of background music (scary, romantic, etc.) on a CD or tape player. Notice how it transforms what you're watching and creates new associations with the event.

Make a video about whatever strikes your fancy. Invent a story, conduct "man-in-the-street" interviews, or film the commonplace—your pet in the backyard, or a family meal from preparation to eating and cleaning up.

Play "smell and tell." Each participant closes his eyes, sniffs an aroma that is held under his nose, and tells what associations come to mind.

Form a band using real or made-up instruments such as pots, pans, a bottle, comb, coffee can, etc.

Assign parts and read a play aloud. Or choose a monologue, and then memorize, prepare, and stage it as an actor would.

🧠 *Singing or reading aloud promotes interaction of the right and left brain and activates normally unused pathways.*

Listen to a piece of music and try to identify the instruments playing. Jazz and blues are good for this exercise. Go to a concert or watch a music video, and then listen to the same piece again on a CD. It's a novel way to "see" with your ears.

9. SPEAK IN SILENCE

Learn sign language. Learning any foreign language is Neurobically stimulating, but learning American Sign Language (ASL) is especially so. Signing requires your hands (and the parts of the cortex that control them) to do something completely new: be responsible for communication. And your visual cortex must learn to associate particular hand positions with meaning, forming links to the parts of the cortex responsible for language and communication. Sign language is challenging, complex, and rich, and requires integrating new types of sensory information to take the place of the usual auditory associations. If you do learn some sign language, you will also be able to communicate with the hearing impaired in a much richer way than when they are reading your lips.

Communicate a thought or idea to someone without using your voice. Playing charades is one fun way to do this, and both actor and guesser benefit.

10. PLAY THE "TEN THING GAME"

Someone hands you an ordinary object. You must use it to demonstrate ten different "things" that the object might be. Example: A fly swatter might be a tennis racket, a golf club, a fan, a baton, a drumstick, a violin, a shovel, a microphone, a baseball bat, or a canoe paddle. In some ways, this game is similar to punning, whereby you reach into your mental sound database and associate a sound/word with something else like it in a humorous way.

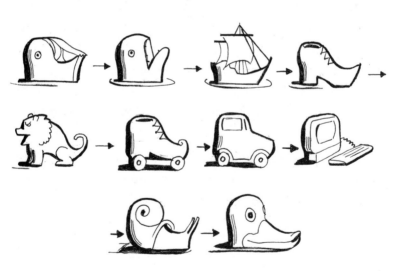

11. PLAY "NAME THAT SOUND"

On an old radio show, contestants would try to identify sounds the host would play for them. You can make up your own after-dinner version of this game. During the week, record sounds on your Walkman from around the house or park or work. Play them back for the family and have each person try to "name that sound." Or buy a sound-effects CD or cassette (there are lots available) and play the game.

12. BRAINATHON

If you already exercise to stay fit, why not give your brain a workout at the same time? Running on a treadmill is not the same as running through a park or your neighborhood. The predictable program of a machine in a gym demands almost nothing of your brain. Walking, jogging, or cycling on a trail or sidewalk opens you up to multisensory experiences with unpredictiblility at every corner…Which way do I go at this intersection? Will that dog come after me? Look out for that kid on the tricycle! So vary your exercise routine by doing it outdoors periodically.

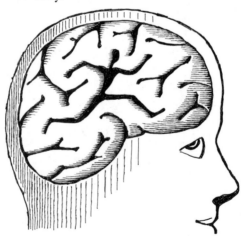

13. PARK ANYWHERE

Parks are designed for leisure activity, especially for exercise of all types.

Try something new like bird-watching or identifying flowers or trees. Fly a kite or go sledding.

Feed the ducks or squirrels (by yourself or with a child). The advantage of Neurobics is that even something small, if unpredictable, is enough to get your brain moving.

Sail a model boat or make one with a simple piece of wood, a stick, and a piece of paper for a sail. Have races!

Settle on a bench, close your eyes, and take in what happens around you. Let your mind free-associate by using the sounds and smells you experience.

14. Start a New Hobby

Hobbies that are most Neurobically stimulating require you to use several different senses in nonroutine ways and to make fine distinctions within one sensory system.

Fly fishing, for example, puts you in a novel sensory environment (a river), requires you to think like a fish and to pay attention to the time of day, the feel of the water, and the types of insects around you. Other examples are archery, photography, woodworking, and cooking.

Master a new gadget such as a computer, video or still camera, telescope, ham radio, musical instrument, Windsurfer, or snowboard.

Learn touch typing. If you still hunt and peck, it slows down your enjoyment of the computer. Practicing touch typing engages the brain in a different way. It offers all the Neurobic benefits of integrating your tactile, spatial, and visual senses without having to be blindfolded.

Build a small model airplane or car while wearing a patch over one eye. Because you lose depth perception, your brain has to rely on new cues. Your sense of touch and spatial skills are required to fit small pieces together.

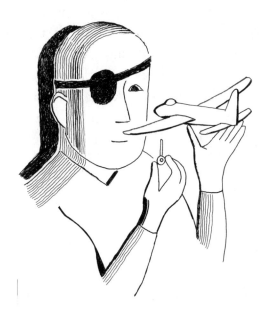

15. GROW A GARDEN, GROW YOUR BRAIN

Whether it's a rooftop flower garden in the middle of a city or a half-acre vegetable plot out in the country, gardening is a good example of a richly Neurobic exercise.

Why? Because you use all your senses in the process: feeling the earth, smelling the fruits and plants, tasting sprigs of herbs. And your brain's planning and spatial abilities are called into action as you decide which plants to put where, the direction of the sun, and how much water is needed. At the end there are potent rewards: fresh, homegrown fruits and vegetables, flowers, or a beautiful yard.

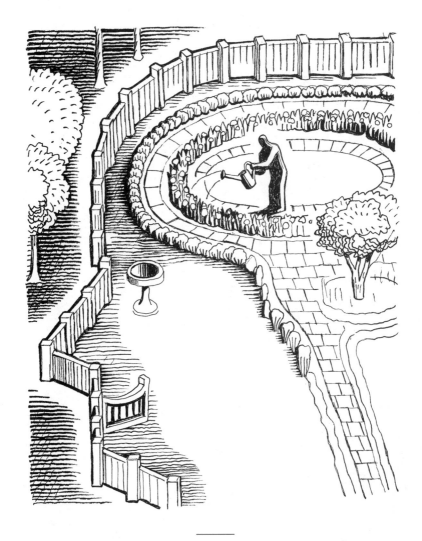

ENDNOTES

Chapter I

1. Dr. Fred Gage of The Salk Institute and researchers at Sahlgrenska University Hospital in Sweden discovered new cell growth in the hippocampus, an area of the brain closely tied to learning and memory, in five patients ages fifty-five to seventy. See the November 1998 issue of *Nature Medicine* for a full report. Using similar techniques, Elizabeth Gould of Princeton University and Bruce S. McEwen at Rockefeller University reported that new cells are constantly being generated in the hippocampus of adult monkeys. (See *Proceedings of the National Academy of Science*, Vol. 95.)

2. Over the past ten years, the issue of whether brain cells die with normal aging has been reexamined by a number of scientists, using much more accurate methods than previously available. The conclusions are clear. Studies such as those by Stephen Buell, Dorothy Flood, and Paul Coleman at the University of Rochester have found that in normal people, even very late in life, the actual number of nerve cells really doesn't change much. So it's likely that most of the nerve cells you had when you were twenty are still very much alive when you're seventy. Even the magnitude of mental decline in normal aging has been overstated: At least 90 percent of the population will age without having to deal with the severe impairments brought about by diseases or strokes.

---

3. In an influential study published in *Science* (Vol. 206) and expanded in *Brain Research* (Vol. 214), Stephen Buell and Paul Coleman found that neurons in the aging human hippocampus (a brain structure critical in learning and memory) actually grew longer dendrites. Interestingly, in the brains of individuals afflicted with Alzheimer's Disease, this growth did not occur. It appears, therefore, that many neurons retain the capacity to grow even late in life.

4. A long series of investigations by Dr. Michael Merzenich at the University of California, San Francisco, has shown the adaptability of connections in the adult brain. For example, in the brains of adult monkeys trained to use certain fingers to get food, the areas of the brain responsible for processing the sense of touch from those fingers gradually took over much larger regions. This means that the brain was able to "rewire" to accomplish something important like getting food, and devoted more "brain horsepower" to the skills required, in this case the sense of touch in certain fingers. Recent findings by Dr. Jon Kaas at Vanderbilt University and Dr. Charles Gilbert at Rockefeller University have shown directly that neurons in the adult brain can actually grow new "wires" to connect to one another.

5. The beneficial effects of neurotrophins have been documented in hundreds of experiments at leading universities throughout the world. In our own experiments at Duke University Medical Center, we (Lawrence C. Katz, A. Kimberley McAllister, and Donald C. Lo) found that adding extra neurotrophins to a neuron almost doubled the size and complexity of the dendrites that branch off the neuron. And since the computing power

of a brain cell is determined by the complexity of its pattern of dendritic branches, this doubling of growth suggests that neurotrophins can literally add more mental horsepower. We were also quite surprised to find that simply adding neurotrophins was not enough. The nerve cells had to be sending or receiving impulses in order to respond to them. The message was clear—adding neurotrophins to *active* neurons made dendrites grow. Conversely, we found that removing neurotrophins made dendrites atrophy (which suggests one reason that brain inactivity leads to mental decline).

6. The first neurotrophin was discovered almost fifty years ago, when two scientists, Rita Levi-Montalcini and Victor Hamburger, working at Washington University in St. Louis, discovered a substance that not only kept certain types of nerve cells alive but also caused them to sprout many new branches. Levi-Montalcini and another scientist, Stanley Cohen, purified this substance, which they named Nerve Growth Factor, or NGF. It turned out that NGF occurred naturally throughout the body but was scarce in the cerebral cortex. NGF was the first member of what became a family of neurotrophins (from the Greek word *trophe*, which, loosely translated, means "to nourish").

In the early 1980s Yves Barde at the Max Planck Institute in Munich, Germany, finally succeeded in purifying a molecule from the brain that behaved just like NGF. Called Brain-Derived Neurotrophic Factor, or BDNF, it was found almost everywhere in the brain, including the cerebral cortex. Neurotrophins have powerful effects on the machinery of the brain. Research by Bai Lu at the National Institutes of Health, Erin Schumann at Caltech, and Tobias Bonhoeffer at the Max Planck Institute in Munich has shown that neurotrophins help increase the strength of connections in the hippocampus, a part of the brain that is critical for learning and memory. Experiments by O. Lindvall and P. Ernfors of University Hospital in Sweden, using animals, suggest that the neurotrophins may protect neurons from damage when parts of the brain undergo a stroke or are damaged by other trauma.

7. Hans Thoenen of the Max Planck Institute in Munich and Christine Gall of the University of California, Irvine, revealed the direct correlation between the production of growth factors and nerve cell activity. Experiments by Anirvan Ghosh and Michael Greenberg at Harvard and Ben Barres at Stanford further showed that this activity-dependent neurotrophin production formed more neural branches and connections, acting, in effect, like a self-fertilizing garden.

8. One example of this kind of stimulation is the patterns of brain activity required to produce a phenomenon called long-term potentiation, or LTP. LTP is a long-lasting change in the strength of synapses between neurons and it has been clearly linked to learning and memory. The same kinds of stimulation that produce LTP also cause increases in the levels of neurotrophins like BDNF.

Chapter II

1. About fifty years ago, a scientist named Karl Lashley trained rats to run a maze for a food reward, and then removed ever larger parts of their cortex to determine when they could no longer "remember" the maze. To his surprise, he found that he could remove about 90 percent of the cortex, and the animals could still find their way! By concluding (wrongly) that only 10 percent of the brain was required for memory to function he missed the more important fact that there are many different forms (representations) of the same memory stored in many different places. When the rats were learning to run the maze, they formed associations among all their senses—they felt, heard, saw, smelled their way through the maze. They had built a net of associations. When one set of associations was destroyed—like those based on vision, for example—they could still rely on their auditory or tactile memories to find their way to the food.

2. And TV viewing is passive. Your sensory systems are involved in only a very limited way, and you are watching someone else perform interesting or exciting activities. But in the brain, watching another person doing something is no substitute for doing it yourself. Indeed, there is direct evidence from animal experiments done by Marion Diamond at University of California, Berkeley, that rats who simply watched other rats playing in an enriched environment derived no brain benefits, while the animals who were actually playing grew larger nerve cells.

3. Michael I. Posner, Marcus E. Raichle, and Steve E. Peterson at Washing-

ton University in St. Louis used functional brain imaging to follow the amount of brain activity in different areas when subjects were asked to come up with a verb to go with a list of new nouns. When first presented with a novel list, large areas of the cortex lit up, showing increased levels of brain activity in several distinct areas of the cortex. After fifteen minutes of practice, when the task had become routine and automatic, activity in those same areas returned to baseline levels. If the subjects were then given a new list, robust activity returned. These researchers also concluded that the brain uses different areas to generate novel responses and automatic (rote) tasks.

4. For a more detailed discussion see: Dr. John Allman, "Tracing the Brain's Pathways for Linking Emotion and Reason," *New York Times,* December 6, 1994.

5. Research by Anthony Damasio and Ralph Adolphs at the University of Iowa has shown how dramatically emotions can enhance memories. The researchers showed a group of people a series of photographs with a simple story about a father taking his daughter to the zoo. Weeks later, when the same people were asked to recount the story, they could recall it only in the vaguest terms. They couldn't remember if it was a son or a daughter…whether she was a blonde or brunette—or even precisely where they were headed. When the scientists changed the emotional quality of the story and pictures to one in which a father takes his daughter to the zoo and she is hit by a car while crossing the road, the memory of the narrative was vastly improved.

6. Long-term studies by groups such as the MacArthur Foundation and the International Longevity Center at Mount Sinai Hospital in New York City reveal that individuals who are most successful at coping with aging and have maintained the best-preserved mental capacities are those who have active social and intellectual networks. Similarly, a three-year study conducted at the University of Southern California showed that people in their seventies who stayed physically and socially active retained their mental faculties much better than individuals who didn't. See *Successful Aging* by Drs. John W. Rowe and Robert L. Kahn for summaries of these and other similar positive findings.

ABOUT THE AUTHORS

Lawrence C. Katz is the James B. Duke Professor of Neurobiology at Duke University Medical Center and an Investigator in the Howard Hughes Medical Institute. A graduate of the University of Chicago, Dr. Katz was a post-doctoral fellow at Rockefeller University, where he worked with Nobel laureate Dr. Torsten Wiesel. He is an internationally recognized expert on the development and function of the mammalian cortex. His recent research focusing on neurotrophins and their effect on nerve cell growth has received widespread recognition in the scientific community and led to the conceptual foundation of this book. Dr. Katz has published over fifty original scientific articles and has received numerous professional awards for his research. In addition to his lab work on the brain, he exercises his brain by flying and fly-fishing. He lives in Durham, North Carolina, with his wife and children.

Manning Rubin, who comes from a long line of writers, has spent most of his career writing in the communications and advertising fields for major firms like Grey and J. Walter

Thompson, as well as running his own movie advertising company. As volunteer Creative Director for The Anti-Defamation League, he has created and consulted on scores of public service ads. A Phi Beta Kappa from the University of Richmond and Johns Hopkins, Manning Rubin is presently stretching his brain as a Senior Creative Supervisor at K2 Design, a leading interactive marketing agency in New York's thriving silicon alley. His book *60 Ways to Relieve Stress in 60 Seconds* was also published by Workman. He lives in New York City with his wife, Jane.

*For news, views, and questions
about keeping your brain active and healthy,
visit: www.keepyourbrainalive.com.*